The Prosperous Personal Trainer: Transform Your Business With High Value Online Programs

TIM DRUMMOND &
PHIL HAWKSWORTH

CONTENTS

1 INTRODUCTION

The bell rang and immediately chaos followed. It was like being in a war zone. You'd have thought I was in Iraq, if there weren't hundreds of guys wearing thousand dollar suits and Franck Muller watches around me. No, this was just the trading floor I worked in the City of London. It was my first day as a trader.

I felt really uncomfortable on that floor. While I was making decent money, I wasn't doing anything that served or benefitted anyone. So eventually I left to become a Personal Trainer. Imagining that I would be helping change loads of people's lives. Boy, was I wrong…

I look back to conversations late at night; my girlfriend asking why we never have the holidays we want. Why we live in rented accommodation. The worst; why I come home from work at 10pm and leave at 6am – never having time to see her.

This had become reality for me. I loved training, nutrition and all of that, but I was questioning my ability to make a living in the fitness industry. Considering looking elsewhere for something more stable.

Frustrated that I was 'self-employed', but completely at the mercy of my clients. Not having any of the freedom I had been promised when I did my PT qualifications.

Stressed about who owed me money, who was away on holiday this month, and if someone was going to leave.

At this stage of my career, I was losing. I like to talk about things in terms of winning and losing. This is what losing looked like, for me.

Does any of this sound familiar?

Welcome

Congratulations on purchasing this book. You have taken the first steps towards more free-time, more income and more enjoyment in your fitness business. Towards becoming a winner in the fitness industry.

Throughout the course of this book we refer to a number of resources which you can download, to action in your fitness business right away. All the resources are available at http://theprosperouspt.com/bonus.

We suggest you go there now, register for free access to everything that you will need to successfully take your fitness business online.

We hope you will not just read this book; think that it sounds good, and then go back to doing exactly what you're doing now. We hope you will go to the resources section at http://theprosperouspt.com/bonus. Download the materials and take action to build a better online fitness business.

When trainers reach out to talk to us, needing help, we lay out two options for them. You can either act and move your life forwards, or you can stay exactly where you are. It is cool whichever you choose to do.

There is no judgement on our part. If you are comfortable and content with your life as it is, you have no reason to change. Just be aware that the choice you make now will affect your business and the rest of your life from this point forwards.

More freedom, income and security are available to you; while you help more people transform their body and life with fitness. We only hope you will be brave enough to take action and do the work to achieve it.

Thankyou,

Tim Drummond & Phil Hawksworth

About This Book

We write with the premise that you are already a good trainer. Someone who is educated and experienced. Someone who cares about their clients and our industry. The fact is, if you didn't care, you wouldn't be reading books to try and improve your business, and your skills. We all know those people who turn up at the gym, have a bit of a laugh and then lark off. We know they're not serious and won't stay in the industry for long.

The fact that you chose to buy and read this book tells us that you are not like that. That you really do care – BUT – you're dissatisfied. You're fed up of working long, unsociable hours; morning, noon and night. Never seeing your family or having any time to yourself. Fed up of having no security and not being able to take time off, because it hits your income too hard. Working with clients that aren't committed, because you need the money.

That's the reality of life for the vast majority of fit-pro's. We have both been there ourselves. This is what drove us to write this book. We could just run off with our secret and have at it, but we remember the suffering that most PT's are stuck in, day to day. We remember what it was like trying to get out of that situation, but not knowing where to look for advice.

Tim remembers back to having difficult conversations with his girlfriend, late at night. Being questioned where is this going? When will business really take off? Why are we still renting accommodation? Why do you work such long hours – would you ever be around when we have kids?

Now remember, most PT's are self-employed. That means the decidedly average wage they make is without all the benefits that most jobs offer. No holiday pay, sick pay or maternity pay. No pension, no health or other benefits. Plus, you probably work a lot more than 40 hours per week.

Fact is, there's more than enough clients to go around. There's a world-wide obesity epidemic! We can teach you this stuff, and know that we are making a difference to people who are in the position that we were in. While at the same time, helping an exponentially greater number of clients transform their bodies than we could ever coach ourselves.

Our Rollercoaster

"So, you're going to tell us this new and better way that we should be running our fitness business. That's cool, but who are you? What has brought you to this place you're at now and why should I listen to you?"

We first met when we were both working at Fitness First in Central London, about 7 years ago. At the time, we were following the typical Personal Training model. Selling 10-blocks of 1-hour training sessions for £500-£600. Always touting for new business on the gym floor and jumping on new members as they came in to the gym. You know how it is.

This was before most trainers even had a website, let alone Facebook ads and all that jazz that people are using now.

We developed together, first as trainers, and then as business owners. A big turning point in our careers came when we attended a PT business event – this was before they were all the rage. We'd never been exposed to this stuff before. As far as we can tell, nobody was really teaching it at that point.

This was our first exposure to learning about marketing, building an email list, selling monthly packages for recurring income and all the things that brought more stability and security to the Personal Training model.

This was great content and stuff that we needed to learn, but it still created more problems. As you become successful, you run out of free time to sell. You will always be capped in how much income you can make, and how many people you can work with at any given time.

As you get busier, you don't even have time for the marketing and business building that got you there in the first place. Causing stagnation and leaving you frustrated.

We had become friends and continued to develop together. Starting to figure the business side of things out a little bit. Unlike many of the other trainers around us, we both had a desire for more. We cared about our clients and our business. We had aspirations to grow and build something bigger. Fitness wasn't just a 'temporary' career.

We were doing well as PT's but that wasn't enough to take us where we wanted to be.

To that end, we started a bootcamp business together. Running short, 30-minute bootcamp sessions for busy women in London. The intention was to grow this model and scale it up. To free ourselves from the time-for-money reality of selling hours of our time to clients in the gym. *The dream.*

We knew that this would create scale and time-freedom. Where we could work on the business and deliver to many people at once. Multiplying our 'hourly-rate' by a factor of 2 or 3. We did this successfully and had a few separate sessions running at a tidy profit. This was only the beginning of our plans.

The long-term vision was to franchise the bootcamp out to other trainers. To scale up and grow nationwide. We would build the brand and manage things centrally. Other trainers could take the concept, the systems we had developed, and roll out in their own area.

We would have a big business that we could systemise and scale. The franchisee gets a ready-made business that they can build quickly. With our support and centralised business management filling in the gaps where a lot of PT's struggle. Namely the business systems and marketing. At least, that was the intention.

Now, at this stage you might be thinking that we didn't make it work, but you will. We used to think like that too, and maybe you will. After all, you've seen a few people have massive success in the fitness industry, right?

We've all had dreams of making it. We all knew lads growing up who had trials and played for the youth teams of professional football clubs, but how many people made it? How many are playing in the Premier League? Or even still playing at all?

A lot of people will get close, but very few ever make it. Our intention is to stack the odds of success in your favour. To help you build an awesome fitness business that your average Sunday League player could make it big with.

£££££ Down the Drain...

Over 3 years of trying, tens of thousands of pounds invested, thousands of hours invested; we never quite got the traction that we were hoping for. We took giant circles around; going from A, right back to A.

What we saw as the way to grow a business, achieve the success and freedom in the fitness industry we desired, relied on so many moving parts. So many things that could – and in our case did – go wrong.

Below we're going to tell you some of the common mistakes and misconceptions that we made, and that Personal Trainers consistently tell us they are making.

This is what we did, and what we see lots of other people doing. It's not to say that it will never work for anybody, but we have not seen it work for many people.

We want you to learn from our mistakes, and the experience of speaking to hundreds of other fit-pros. Save yourself tens of thousands of pounds, years of your life and not have to learn the hard way. Trust us, it will be better that way.

There is a much better way to build a business, which we will explain as the book progresses.

Here's where you might be at with your thinking right now, and why that might be a mistake:

> You need an amazing website, and SEO/Google will bring you loads of clients.

We went through 3 different websites in our business, over the course of 3-4 years. Each one an upgrade on the last, costing more money and taking more time to build.

I spoke to a girl recently who had paid a well-known 'expert' for 9 months, was paying him a lot of money, and she still didn't have a finished website. This mirrors our experience when we laid out thousands for a high-end, bespoke website which took a similar amount of time.

Spending all this time trying to get it right. Writing and re-writing the copy, tweaking design and obsessing about logos is a great way to keep you procrastinating in the same place you are now. Too much thinking goes into this, and not enough time, effort and money actually *doing* anything.

Of course, the other option is to build your own website. Great if you are a qualified web designer. Assuming that you're not, we usually see it taking forever, being frustrating and overwhelming. Leading to most people giving up and never finishing it. Wasting a lot of time in the process. Then paying for a pro to do it in the end anyway.

Now when it comes to SEO, it does bring you leads, and works great for local PT. Consider the search behaviour of potential customers. They will be searching for "Personal Trainer in London". If you are ranking for that term, you will be found.

Nobody is searching for "online Personal Trainer". They are aware of the problem they have, but are not aware that an online trainer is a viable solution. The market is there, but they are not actively searching for you. This will make more sense as you read on.

Even SEO only works some of the time. For starters, it depends heavily on where you are based. If you are in a very competitive market, there will be lots of people already spending lots of time and money to get the best rankings.

We see many people come back a year later to their web designer and complain that their SEO isn't working. Why? It's because they're not consistently creating content and engaging on social media, which are the most important factors for Google's latest algorithm.

We had an SEO person do our website – this was back when it was much easier to rank in Google than it is now, and was based mostly on keywords – and we did get leads from it. However, if you have a website you probably have the experience of *finally* getting a lead in, after weeks of waiting. You're excited and email them back immediately; only to never hear from them again.

Leads coming from your website seem to disappear off the face of the earth much more commonly than leads coming from elsewhere.

We're not against websites. A website offers some good benefits, but it's like if I ask a fit-pro about Weight Watchers. Most will agree that it has *some* good parts, and it helps *some* people in *some* ways, but it's not the *best* way to do things.

When This Happens… When That Happens…

Many Personal Trainers think they cannot get online clients because they don't have a big profile or reputation. You might be well-known locally, but have no presence online.

We thought that getting in national media was a great way to build a big profile and position ourselves as the best in the eyes of the public. Bringing in loads of leads in the process.

The fact is, you can get high-paying clients, even if nobody knows who you are. We were worse than most people for thinking that we couldn't succeed without a big profile. We spent thousands of pounds every month getting into magazines and newspapers.

Truth is, that wasn't the real problem. Our real problem was that we didn't have the right offer, or enough leads coming in. We thought media would bring in lots of leads, but it didn't.

Even if it had, without the right offer it would have been useless anyway.

Our first big piece of coverage came out in *The Sun*, right around Christmas. I was out for Christmas drinks with the guys from the gym when it was released. This was exciting. This was going to be when we took off for sure. All our friends congratulated us, we were on such a high. I remember proudly posting it on Facebook, and telling my parents about it.

This was it – we had 'made it' now. I went back home that Christmas. All my old friends, who were still just finishing university and starting their careers were so impressed. They thought I must be killing it.

We never "killed it" from the coverage.

This "it will take off when… [insert every new shiny object we were chasing]" became a central tenant of where our business was. It was always going to happen when "the next thing" came off.

Our egos were getting a good stroking from this 'fame', and we were building that all important 'know, like and trust' with our market, like all the marketing experts told us. Not a bad thing, but there are much better ways to build trust, help more clients and add money to the bank, which we go into detail on later.

The Wrong Offer

> If you're not getting leads and clients, you think it is a problem with your website, or lack of exposure.

You can write and re-write, tweak and re-tweak your website as much as you want. If you are not getting the fundamental offer right, it doesn't matter how you dress it up.

When we say 'the offer', we mean the proposition of what we give to clients. The offer that we are making them in exchange for their time and money.

In our bootcamp business the thing we were presenting to them was just not compelling enough for them to get excited about and committed to it. It was too bland. Too samey. Every fitness person ever has said the same thing.

Imagine that you own a restaurant. You see someone walking down the street who is obviously hungry. Visibly starving.

Meanwhile, you have a fat, juicy steak sizzling away on the grill. You can smell it, taste it in the air. You're drooling like a dog, excitedly waiting for this customer to come in and eat your steak. Why wouldn't they right? It's a no-brainer.

You have recognised their problem – hunger, and you have the solution – your steak.

Yet that person is *never* going to respond to your offer. Why?

They're vegan.

No matter how you dress up your steak, how many ways you communicate it, how much social proof you have of other people saying they love your steak, how satisfying it looks, you will never sell a steak to this person.

That is what we mean by the 'wrong offer'. They want the outcome (to no longer be hungry) but they're simply not in the market for a steak. Your solution is irrelevant to them.

Back to fitness – your offer is working out in the gym, training for an hour to lose weight. Maybe you'll "beast them", or maybe you'll teach them complex "functional fat-burning routines".

Really, what most people want is simple, fast and easy. They don't like the sound of hard work, or anything that brings them too far out of their comfort zone.

They want to lose weight in a manageable, easy way that doesn't make them too uncomfortable. They want to feel confident in their body, to wear their favourite outfit that hasn't fit for years, and go out on the dating market, comfortable in their body, believing that they are attractive.

You know the problem (their body) and the solution (losing weight) but your offer of how to do it is not resonating with their desire.

The right offer will meet people where they are with their thinking, communicate in their language and offer the solution that they *think* they need.

The Wrong Business Model

> Just getting people in the door, even if it's for free, will give me the exposure I need to grow.

We were trying to build our business from the bottom up. Get a high volume of low paying clients. In hindsight, the Tesla Motors model of starting at the top with a small number of high value clients, and then filtering down into a mass market offer, is a much better business.

The Tesla Model

The tesla business model is to start off with a premium priced offering that has a high profit margin.

This can be produced in small numbers, while yielding a good profit, which is then re-invested back into expansion. The more high-priced cars they sell, the more profit they have, to invest in further infrastructure, staff, systems, etc. to produce more cars and thus more profits.

Eventually they bring out mid-market options that have been honed with the technology and engineering skills built making the premium models. This is paid for with the profits from the premium offers and eventually they produce a mass market car.

All while remaining profitable, not having to take on the risk of financing a mass market offering to begin with, that can so easily fail.

You can do the same with a premium high-priced coaching model, and if you so choose, eventually go mass market with books, membership sites, group training, etc.

Instead of a long period of setting up, and high start-up cost, you can finance it all with the profits from your premium offers.

It gives the security of money in the bank, consistent cashflow and ensures that you are generating revenue as quickly as possible.

> Personal Trainers want to scale and systemise their business. To get other trainers doing their sessions, or open their own training studio. That's a pretty common aspiration in the fitness industry.

The problem is, people are saying this when they don't even have enough clients themselves. How are you going to fill sessions up for someone else, when you can't even fill your own sessions?

Assuming you do have enough clients to make this work, it has a whole other set of problems that every studio owner we speak to mentions. Trainers will start stealing your clients. Trainers will let you down. Not turn up, not do a good job, not be professional, etc.

It's easy to say that you won't employ those types of trainers, but who would you employ? Think about it, would you work for someone else?

How are you going to find good, qualified, professional trainers that will work for a fraction of the money they could get on their own?

You're either going to get people new to the industry who want to learn from you, but will soon leave when they have done so. Possibly taking their clients with them. Or you're going to get people who just don't care, don't put in the effort or otherwise could not succeed on their own.

It's a tough model to make work.

Social Media

> I can get clients from social media though?

Everyone and their Grandma is on social media nowadays. It can be a great source of clients, but are you already getting clients directly from social media right now?

Most trainers we speak to spend a lot of time on social media, for little to no reward.

The Facebook business page gets tiny interaction if you're not paying for boosting. You can get people into a free group, but still there is no interaction and nobody goes on to buy anything.

Of course, you can run ads, but Facebook are consistently moving the goalposts, making life difficult for fit-pros. You think you have it figured out eventually, then they go and change the rules and you're back to not getting your ad approved.

Maybe you have followers on Instagram, Twitter or somewhere else and spend hours every day curating posts. Having an audience is a good start, but hardly anybody is getting clients or making any money from their audience.

Followers and likes do not pay the bills.

One of Tim's clients had 15,000 Instagram followers, but absolutely no idea how to make money with that asset. Making money on social media is like teenage sex; everyone says they are doing it, most aren't and those who are, are doing it badly.

The return on the time invested is less than you'd get working at McDonald's. That's assuming you can even maintain doing it. So many simply get overwhelmed and quit their social media strategy after a couple of weeks, without any positive returns.

Using Free or Cheap Offers to Get People in The Door

I just need exposure to more people, right?

We used Groupon to fill up our classes with people, assuming that after the first (very cheap) month was over, they would stay on at full price.

Nowadays people are doing it with free or low priced trials, free Facebook groups and trying to upsell clients through to bigger packages. Unfortunately, for the most part someone who is willing to pay £7 for a Facebook group is not the same person who is going to pay hundreds or thousands for a personal transformation.

No matter how you dress it up, most of these people are never going to pay you anything, or anything further than the tiny amount they begin on. Meanwhile, these are the people who ask the most stupid questions and expect everything to be free.

My Brand Needs Work!

> People obsess over logos, names, changing the look of their website or printing business cards.

Not just personal trainers, it's a commonality in most small-scale entrepreneurs who will spend time doing anything apart from marketing and selling their products/services.

We had our website redesigned 3 times, each at significant cost and rebranded the whole business once. We lost months of time while we were hamstrung with no brand or web presence, which meant we did next to no marketing.

This was one of our worst "when this happens" moments. We put everything on this new brand, while still not having a plan for how we were going to generate clients. The fact is, a shiny logo does not cause all your dream clients to come knocking your door down.

The amount of times we said, "it doesn't matter what's happening now. We're putting everything in place for the future. It's all about the long term!" - sheesh.

We were delusional, but everyone thought we were really successful. We looked the part, but had nothing to back it up.

We eventually closed that business because it wasn't going anywhere. Having made just about every mistake in the book along the way.

Still with us?

Good. Now, that's a pretty epic tale in failure. Perhaps it's arrogant to look back in hindsight and say that, knowing what we know now, we would have made it successful. However, the one theme that was going on throughout the whole business, was this: *distraction.*

This is where our tale of woe becomes relevant for you.

We did everything and anything under the sun, apart from the one thing that we needed to do.

I heard a quote the other day, it's from Michael Masterson in the book 'Ready, Fire, Aim'. The quote goes something like this;

"The only thing that matters from 0 – 1 million dollars' revenue, is sales".

If we had just generated leads and sold, without a website, without fancy branding, without social media, without PR, without a book and without £3,000 videos – we would probably have been successful.

Of course, that stuff does need to come later to make a business like that scale. Our business model had a low average customer value, so we would need lots of customers. That means you cannot do all the delivery yourself. You're going to need help.

This is why we conclude now that it was a bad business model. Too many moving parts. Too many things that can go wrong. Too much reliance on other people who are not invested enough in the business that they can be relied upon.

2 BROKEN BUSINESS MODEL = BROKEN BUSINESS

That business required reaching a critical mass where it would start to grow outside of our hustle. In hindsight, we were unlikely to ever get there.

A better model, is one that has a high average customer value. In which you can do the hustling to get things moving, and it is feasible and scalable, because you only need a few clients who are easy to find and easy to manage. We weren't joking when we said it's the same amount of work to get a high-paying client, as it is to get a low-paying client. It's probably less, for reasons we will explore later in the book.

Average Customer Value

Average customer value is the average amount of money a customer will spend with you, over their lifetime.

Some clients or customers will make only one transaction, while others will stay with you for years and continue to buy, month after month. Some businesses have high-value transactions, while others have low-value transactions.

The higher the average customer value, the less customers you need to achieve your revenue goals. To achieve a high average customer value, you need either a high price point, or long time retention. Preferably both!

In a service business it's generally much easier to acquire and manage a smaller number of high-value customers than to try and deal with lots of low-value customers.

Tim's mentorship client Adam was able to upsell some £30 per hour in-person clients in to a £2k 12-week program, and then a year- long £8k program online. Hugely increasing the value of those customers.

It might not be sexy, but the less moving parts there are in a business, the easier it is. Complicated funnels are the problem, not the solution. Contrary to what most people think, simplicity is important.

It's like coaching a client, you don't tell them every single thing you've learnt since day one of PT School. All the courses you've studied, every book you've read. You simplify it and give them only what they need to know.

You need to know the million and one things that might affect their weight loss, but you only need to tell them the one or two big things that are going to make all the difference. Apply simplicity in your business by understanding the complexity, and then prioritising effectively.

It's easy to be busy as a Personal Trainer working in a gym, because it is simple. Client joins gym, you talk to them, they train with you. That's all there is to it – literally nothing else needs to happen. You just rinse and repeat talking to people in the gym, and then training those people. Simplicity!

The problem with that model, is when you run out of hours. It doesn't scale well, you don't make enough money, but it at least works easily, to make you a living income; if not much more than that.

Anyway, the next phase; after that business failed is when we went our separate ways business wise and both actually started making progress.

We'd learnt a lot, as you do, from failing in business. The biggest thing that we changed was seeking help. We'd been arrogant before, thinking that we knew how to do it ourselves.

Getting Help

Looking back now, if we had just paid £2,000 for a day with a top business coach, who knew how to build a business (and listened to them), we would have:

1) Saved 10's of thousands in money spent on all the things we wasted it on.

2) Saved us years of time, effort and stress

3) Not to mention the opportunity cost of losing two years of making the money we make now, having the freedom and lifestyle that we currently enjoy.

We both invested in help from coaches and mentors, and that really helped us to move forwards.

To cut away all the distraction and go back to a simple, effective business model that works. We both knew that Personal Training wasn't going to take us where we wanted to be.

Phil wanted to be free to travel the world; not tied to a location or schedule. To be able to set up in a coffee shop in Rio de Janeiro or Bali, and do his work from there.

Tim wanted to earn enough to buy a house, and eventually, to build his own house. Where he can start a family, with the security of plenty of money coming in to support them.

The answer to both, was to work online. If you want freedom and if you want to scale your earning up, online is the best place to do it in the fitness industry.

We will explore exactly what the new business model looks like later in the book. First, we need to address where the current model – the Personal Training model – is failing you. Leaving you burnt out and stuck. It's important to understand this, because when you do, it indicates what you should do instead.

Listen, the model works just fine if you're happy earning £20,000 per year – maybe £30,000 in London. If you're happy with that, put this book down right now and go find *another* client, deliver *more* sessions.

Seriously, this isn't us being condescending. We mean it, because if you're happy with that, who are we to tell you different?

Just hope that you don't ever get sick…
Or ever want to go on holiday…
Or ever get injured…
Or have a partner that wants to see you now and then…
Or kids you'd like to see grow up.

Knowing the pitfalls of the status quo is the first part of making a positive change. If you think that Personal Training is OK. If you're content to sell your time for money, to work long and unsociable hours, and never make a lot of money, then you are not going to be motivated to make the changes required.

The changes are not 'hard'. The business model is incredibly simple, and even less work than Personal Training. However, it will be uncomfortable. You will have to do things that you probably don't like doing. To succeed, you need to get out of your comfort zone and put yourself out there. To do the one or two things that will move you forwards, despite the fear and doubt you might suffer. In this sense, it is challenging.

Case Study: Joe

Joe was a PT working in a budget box gym in Portsmouth. Never charging more than £250 for 10 sessions, after 5 years in the industry.

He was making £3k/month by working 14 hour days. 34 paid hours per week. Never at home, didn't ever spend time with his girlfriend, missing out on his social life. Didn't have time to really offer a good service, write programs and be consistent with his service to all of his clients.

Joe had a 1-week break in August and that was the first time he had taken time off for a full year. This was when he realised how tired he was, how his own training was suffering and that he needed to do something different.

Joe wanted to get to £8k/month. They want to have kids at some point, and his girlfriend wants to go part time at work. Plus, Joe wants free time to do his own training, travel more and enjoy his social life while he is young.

In the first 5 weeks of coming on board in Tim's mentorship Joe made 4 online sales. The first sale was to a current client, upsold to the online program. Without needing a website, big email list or Facebook ads. Joe says this was the easiest sale he ever made. Sitting down together with his client, they had a deeper conversation than he'd had in 2 years with that client. They'd never got that much depth before.

The client immediately opened up and was on board. No price objection and signed up there and then. The client was extremely grateful for this extra level of service, and the feeling of being listened to and understood that came from Joe having that conversation with them.

Currently Joe is bringing down his 1-1 hours. He has the money to get rid of some clients he doesn't want to work with, and focus only on the committed ones he loves to train. The other clients can be passed to other trainers, and Joe can offer the higher level of service and excellence that he wants to the select clients who are a perfect fit for what he does.

Why the Personal Training Model is Failing You, & Where the Future Lies

Personal Training is a young industry that is still finding its feet. The industry that we work in is probably about the same age as you or I. Maybe even younger. The point is, the fitness industry is still finding its feet and learning how to get on in the world.

It changes extremely quickly, and is changing often. New concepts are introduced, and the consensus of people in the industry shifts to a new paradigm. There's currently an explosion of new people coming in to the industry. It has never been easier, faster or cheaper to become a Personal Trainer.

You could look at this as a good thing – because it shows the demand for fitness is growing and people are waking up to, and trying to fix, the obesity epidemic. Likewise, you could look at it as a bad thing – an already competitive industry is becoming more so, while the barrier to entry decreases and overall quality of service possibly follows it.

Either way, opinion on the matter doesn't matter so much as recognising that a change is happening. Whether you're happy about it or not, you need to be on board with it, or risk being left behind. We think that throughout this book we will make the argument that this change is a good thing, for you.

Whether it is good for the industry as a whole is up for debate, but that's not the topic of this book. We are focused on helping you to have the business and lifestyle that you desire, in the new Personal Training economy.

Why the Old Model of Personal Training Sucks for You

"So, why is the old model of Personal Training not working? What are some of the problems with it?"

The biggest problem that we hear time and time again, when we speak to trainers, is that even when you are 'successful' in the Personal Training model, it's not offering the lifestyle and freedom that you desire. This doesn't sit well, if you are at the top of your field, you should be rewarded for it.

Problem with Personal Training – and this is true of many service businesses – is that 'success' equals working more. More clients, more hours, more time in the gym, more diet plans to write, more emails and texts to respond to.

You're selling your time and to make a decent - but still pretty modest - amount of money, you end up selling almost all your time.

Going home at the end of the day, after 12 hours in the gym, you're too exhausted to do anything for yourself. You don't see much of your family or friends.

If you don't have a family yet, you won't know what this is like. A guy once said to me; all that he wants from his business, is to be able to take the evening off to take his lad to football training.

He can't, because he's scared of losing the income and not being able to pay the bills. He knows he's letting his son down, but hopes his lad will understand. I asked him if he felt his son does, and he solemnly said "no…".

Even your training and eating, the very things that you are supposed to be the model of excellence for, take a hit. You don't have enough time to train properly, or to cook. Over time, this takes its toll on your physique, your energy and your health. Suddenly you're not quite in the shape you used to be, despite having more knowledge and experience in the fitness world. You just don't have the time to implement it yourself!

Worse still, it takes its toll on you mentally, and suddenly you're not quite as in love with your work as you once were.

So…?

Most PT's think the answer to this is getting more leads, more clients. Maybe putting their prices up £5-10.

Imagine you're driving along a road, and you spot that there's a cliff 100m in front of you. Continuing this same business model – adding *more* fuel to the fire is like pressing hard on the accelerator. You're just going to drive off the cliff quicker.

If the volume game - selling as many hours of your life as possible - isn't going to work for you, you need to do a hard-left turn and avoid the cliff. You need to change business model, to something that is sustainable and has the room to grow without you flying off a cliff when you inevitably burn out.

Of course, you could work less hours, but that's not a solution, because you will be earning less money. Even while you're very busy and doing well for a Personal Trainer, honestly, it's not exactly getting the bank manager excited to meet you. You need all the money you are bringing in and then some. Taking a pay cut for an easier life is not an option.

What other options are out there?

You could charge more for your sessions, but you're already at or near the limit. Maybe increasing it £5-10 over time, but that's not going to move the needle. In fact, it's barely going to keep up with increasing gym rent and travel costs anyway. Inflation and cost of living have been increasing faster than Personal Trainer's income for the last few years.

Clients are just not going to pay much more than they already are. There's a 'going rate' in your area, and once you're at the top of it, that's pretty much your limit. Most people don't have the luxury of living down the road from a Russian Oligarch who can throw silly money at them for training.

When we were both doing the old model of Personal Training, in the financial district and most affluent areas of central London, we charged top rates in that market. Still, we weren't making significantly more than the average successful PT. Training high-flying executives, Hedge Fund owners and a few celebrities still didn't put us in the position to make a good living from Personal Training.

It might have felt good for our egos. Being at the top of the industry and interacting with highly successful people, but the daily grind was the same. To be honest, for Phil, at the age of 23, it was good money. Better than university graduate jobs – but it would still have been the same – and much less impressive – in 20 years' time, had we continued that path.

"Should I put my prices up?", you're thinking.

Well, probably yes. If you're good. If you get results and care about your clients, you should push the boat and charge as much as you can.
That's not the answer though. You will creep an inch or two closer to that

glass ceiling, but you're still only on the first floor. You're still going to end up banging your head.

Why bother scrapping to inch your way up? A better business model will whisk you straight up to the penthouse in a private elevator.

Not Sure About Letting Go of the Old Model?

Tell me if this sounds like you...

You get up in the dark to go train clients before they go to the office. It's probably cold and wet outside. You spend all day in the gym and you're still there, waiting, when the office workers stream out of the office at the end of the day. They don't care that you've been in the gym for 10+ hours already, they still expect the same level of energy and enthusiasm; and why shouldn't they? They're paying the same rates after all.

When you finally get out of the gym, again, it's dark. I hope you're supplementing your Vitamin D?

This is what every day is like. Even when you go home, you're never really 'off the clock'. You don't get to check out of work, like people with normal jobs, and relax down the pub. You have emails, texts to reply to. Programs to write and money to chase up. Not forgetting Fred who hasn't turned up for his last 3 training sessions and needs some variation of support/encouragement/scolding.

Then you need to update your status on 4 different social media platforms, and send an email to your list. You haven't blogged for a couple of weeks, but you just don't have the time or energy right now.

No Escape...

I remember going on holiday to Egypt a few years ago. I went the week before Christmas, precisely because the gym was quiet, and clients were starting to fall off for the Christmas break. I finally felt like I could go away, and not feel guilty that I was letting my clients down.

I'd not taken a holiday in almost 2 years. How can you? Clients rely on you to be there; they've paid for their sessions. They're going to want money back if you're not there to train them.

You're going to spend money on the holiday, earn no money because you aren't working. You're still paying gym rent, even though you're not there, and some of your clients will want refunding for missed sessions. Going on holiday essentially costs 3 times as much as the cost of the holiday, when you consider the lost earnings, continued expenses and everything else. Anyway, first holiday in 2 years. I rock up on the beach in Dahab – one of the top 3 diving spots in the world. Beautiful coral reef that rivals the Great Barrier Reef any day. Of course, laying on the beach the *first day*, I get sick.

I've been so stressed and worn down. Not sleeping enough; early mornings, late nights. No time off and no escape from the grind. As soon as my body senses a bit of relaxation, it immediately proceeds to get sick. I'd probably been carrying an infection for weeks. Too doped up on adrenaline for my body to feel comfortable fighting it off.

If you've ever dived, you will know that it doesn't work if you're blocked up. You can't breathe and they won't let you go. So, my week diving one of the world's best reefs became a week laying on the beach, snot running out of my nose, coughing and spluttering on to my book.

Not quite the holiday I had in mind.

Case Study: Owen

When Owen first came to me, he was working 60-hour weeks. Starting at 6am and finishing with clients at 9pm. He never had evenings off and hadn't taken a holiday in over 4 years. He was earning money, but he was a slave to his business. He had no freedom and was on a fast-track to burnout.

He wanted to be able to go online full time, so he could travel more. He wanted to earn more money, to better provide for his family, and was hoping to get engaged to his girlfriend. He'd not had the easiest upbringing and wanted to ensure he provided a better platform for his kids – this desire is what got him through 60-hour weeks for so long.

He'd added online training about 18 months prior, but it wasn't working. He struggled to get leads and was frustrated with people emailing their interest and then dropping off.

Owen needed help with his business model to attract the right clients. Then learning how to deliver a superior service for his online clients.

Since starting in my mentorship he has sold on average 4 clients per month (at $3k). No longer stressing about where the next dollar is coming from, or how to provide a good service to online clients. He's getting great results and happily posting all the before & after photos on Facebook.

Plus, he has even upsold one of his clients into a year-long program for $10,000.

Adding $12,000 of online income to his existing in person income took his earnings over $20,000 per month. He kept some high-paying in person clients because he enjoys training them, but now has the freedom to choose his hours.

It took 5 weeks to get the first sale, but that confidence opened the floodgates and he made 3 sales in just 6 days. That's $9,000 cash sitting in his bank account, all paid up front.

With the money he's making, and the confidence that it isn't all going to fall apart, he has not only proposed to his girlfriend, but did so with a huge diamond ring. Something he never thought he could have done just a few months earlier.

What else?

Hey, we're just getting warmed up. Not that we want this to be a pity party, but we need to look at what happens when you're not just following the old model, but - much worse - you're actually succeeding.

It's too easy to just accept it as the everyday reality, and not expect that there is scope for things to be better. Well guess what… there is. We are going to make damn sure that you can see that by the end of this book.

Over the years too many great trainers have left the industry because they're worn out, disillusioned and feel that it is not going anywhere. It's an emotionally taxing job. People in the outside world don't realise how tiring it can be, having all your clients coming in, back to back, to unload their emotional problems on you, while you're trying to do a set of squats. We're not therapists, after all, as much as it might feel like we are at times.

Funny thing is, the more clients we have, the more 'successful' we are, the worse our service gets. We have less time to give to each client outside of the contact time – planning sessions, supporting them and keeping them accountable. The more people we have to keep up with, the harder it is to keep up.

Not to mention, our overall energy level and enthusiasm, showing up every hour of every day, in a good mood.

It's a bad thing when this starts to affect the service you give to clients, but it's a deal breaker when it starts affecting your family. Coming home late, getting up early, never having the time to give to your relationship, things start to drift apart.

If you've got kids, you are in a real catch 22 situation. You can go and work the long hours required to earn the money and provide a good life for them. Or you can spend time with them, seeing them grow up, reading to them at night, playing in the park.

Choose one, because you're going to struggle to do both.

Busted!

Have you ever been caught watching the clock or checking texts by a client? It feels awful. They know you're not engaged and excited to be there with them. Even when it's innocent. You're reading a text from your next client, who is asking if they can re-arrange their session; it's still detracting from the client stood in front of you right now.

And what about those clients who just don't do what you say. You know the ones. You're a great trainer and get amazing results with most of your clients...but there's always a few who just don't do what you say. They don't follow your advice and perhaps worse, they lie to you about it. Maybe they're lying to themselves too; not doing it knowingly. Either way, it doesn't matter. Fact is, they're not getting the outcomes that they want and are paying for.

These clients are typically the ones who most need the help as well. They seem like they're in the most desperate situation, but will not follow through on what they need to do to get out of it!

Ever had a client who's been with you for 2 years, and is pretty much the same weight as they were when they started - not cool, right?

Personal Training suddenly starts to feel like a dreaded j-o-b. You're going through the motions. Turning up to earn your pay check. That is not why you got in to the industry! I know it, because I've done it myself.

Dread...

After enough time banging your head against the wall with certain clients, you simply start to dread seeing them. A couple of sessions per week starts draining 50% of your energy. That hour ruins your whole afternoon, and Wednesday lunch is feeling like Friday night.

You're better than that though. You *are* good at what you do. You have extensive knowledge and experience. You care and want to be known as someone who excels with all their clients. Someone who really helps people to transform their bodies and lives. If only all your clients would do what you said!

When I was training the owner of a big, successful hedge fund, I really thought I had made it. He has more money than sense (literally). He's a big guy, clearly has been so focused on work that he has totally neglected his body. Plus, having that much money, he is attractive to a certain kind of woman, despite not being in the best of shape, so he doesn't even have that incentive.

Well, I have never known a client to be such hard work. Re-arranging – no joke – over 50% of his sessions at the last minute (and paying a re-arrangement fee that is double what most trainers charge for their sessions).

He was paying me a large amount of money, but he owned me. I daren't challenge him too much.

I'm not proud of this, but he was paying me so much money that I was intimidated. I feared losing him as a client, because he was such a big percentage of my income.

He never took it seriously. I think spending the money and (occasionally) turning up at the gym let him kid himself that he was doing something about his weight. Without having to actually make, or even consider making, the changes he needed to. I told myself that it was OK. He's better off training sometimes than not at all. He'll be fitter and healthier, even if he has only lost a couple of pounds.

Fast forward a year: after I'd become successful online and was making more than enough money, I had another big money in-person client.

(By the way; that's a choice that you have, you can still work with people offline if you choose to. *If you choose to*).

Anyway, this guy came from opulent wealth. He'd never wanted for anything and was used to everyone around him being 'yes men'. He'd tried loads of different PT's to get in shape, including being at the most expensive gym in the UK (just the price of membership is eye-watering).

I could get phenomenal results with this guy, when nobody else ever had, because from day 1 I could maintain the power in the relationship. I didn't become another 'yes man', like I would have in the past. I set the boundaries, told him what was acceptable and what wasn't. Having that authority lead to him actually following through with the things he needed to do.

In week 1, he had rocked up late once or twice, and I told him it wasn't good enough. I called him out and told him that he either takes this seriously and does as he is told, or I will refund his money and he can clear off. (He was paying me what most PT's earn in 6 months).

He respected this, nobody had ever been honest with him before about what needed to happen to change his body. I had the security to do this – to really serve this guy – because of the money in the bank, and system to generate more, online.

He still messages me sometimes, years later, just to say thank you and update me on his progress. Being secure online allowed me to serve my offline clients at the highest level.

The Final Nail in the Coffin for a Successful PT

The ironic thing of being busy and successful in the old model of Personal Training, is that you have no free time to work on your business. You have visions of doing things online, having a studio or running a retreat. You just do not have any free time, or energy, to make it happen.

On top of this, you don't even have the time to find new clients. It only takes 1 or 2 regular clients leaving and suddenly there's a big hole in your income, with no prospects ready to fill it. You haven't had the time to speak to anyone or find new clients, because every hour of the day is taken up with your existing clients.

Meanwhile, the freshly qualified trainer who did his PT course in 3 weekends last month is undercutting your prices and scooping up all the available new business. How has this guy got 30 hours of PT already? He's barely beyond being a danger to his clients.

Not to hate on the guy, I'm sure he is educating himself and wants to get better, but he doesn't have the skills and experience to really help his clients – yet he is picking up business like I don't know what.

Of course, undercutting prices will get him moving, but soon he will be in the same situation as you – too busy, no time or energy – AND he won't even be making a lot of money, because his packages are too cheap.

Even when things are going well, there's this sense of uneasiness that Personal Training doesn't lead anywhere. I remember when I started out, the first year was a grind. I struggled and was broke for a while as I built my client base up.

Once I got established and had figured out how to attract and keep clients, it was pretty awesome for a year or so. I was free to focus on educating myself and becoming a better trainer. But by the end of that second year, I was starting to question what happens next.

Where do I go from here? I'm already working all the hours that I want to work. I've put up my prices to be more expensive than anyone else in my gym. I just don't see myself selling hours of my time for the rest of my life. I want more than that.

I wanted to have the freedom to travel and work from anywhere in the world – that was my most pressing goal. It's OK to work all the time, when you're in your early twenties and just starting out.

What about when you want to have kids? You've probably bought a house, which means you must keep earning what you're making, to pay the mortgage; but working 10-12 hour days means you will never see your children grow up. You can't work less, but you can't find more free time either. It's a lose-lose situation.

Then what? You're the '40-year-old PT' and still putting in the grind, walking the gym floor? That's not what I have in mind, that's for sure.

The Scaling Problem

Personal Training (and most service-based businesses) don't scale. You cannot run the business without directly selling your time, because you are the product. Having your own studio or training company is possible of course, but the investment and risk are huge. You're going to end up working twice as much to get it off the ground. Invest thousands, go in to lots of debt, and take on a lot of risk.

Everyone I know who has bootstrapped their own studio (as opposed to having investment) has kept it afloat from the money they bring in from their own clients – so there is no respite there – until it became established and the business started making money of its own, you're going to be working your ass off more than ever.

It does work, but it's high-risk, incredibly hard work, and with all the costs and overheads, not even very profitable *if* you do succeed, against the odds.

A friend of ours who owns 3 successful training studios in London, with a team of about 30 trainers says that if he knew what he knows now at the beginning, he would never have gone that route.

Thankfully, we are now both in the position that we want to be in, and neither of us are putting in the daily grind, being in the gym from 5am until 8pm.

Phil travels the world freely and is writing this from a coffee shop in Thailand. Tim just bought his first home and works from there for a few hours a day, with his new puppy Horatio, earning six-figures doing so.

How did we get in this position?

The first thing that we realized, a long time ago, was that the Personal Training model was broken. It was simply never going to create the kind of business and life that either of us desired. More than that, it wasn't going to allow all the great trainers that we know, who excel in what they do and care about their clients, to ever be rewarded as they deserve.

Personal Training Is Broken

The problem with the industry, on a meta scale, is that it is selling the wrong thing. Clients do not want a Personal Trainer!

Controversial, I know. Let me explain. A client has a problem that they are unhappy with:

They're overweight, sick and lacking confidence. Because of this they are single, coming up to 35, have no children, don't ever go on dates, and fear that this will never change.

The client has a desire that they want to achieve:

They want to be slim, healthy and feeling good in their body. They want the confidence to go out and meet someone, to be able to have children and fulfill a bigger life purpose.

Their problem is not lack of a Personal Trainer, and their greatest desire is not to have someone stand next to them, counting their reps and shouting words of encouragement. No. The client wants to achieve the outcome; to change their body. *Changing their body will change their life*, by the way.

Nobody Wants Your Amazing List of Features

One of the 'rules' of marketing is that people do not want to buy your product and all its fancy features – they simply don't care. They want to buy the solution to their problem, the benefits to them. This is the only thing they care about.

"Don't sell me a drill bit; sell me the picture frame hanging from the hole in the wall".

Benefits, Not Features

Features are the component parts of your service; such as training 3x per week, a diet plan, email support.

Features are what allow you to deliver the service, and are important in that sense, but they are not compelling. Every Personal Trainer does the same things and nobody is going to choose to work with you for these reasons.

Benefits are the outcome the client gets from your service; such as losing weight, having more confidence, getting big guns that impress the girls.

Benefits are what people are really buying, and what you should express in your presentation of what you do.

To make sure you get this right, use the words "so that". What follows will be the benefit.

Example:

Bespoke diet plan **so that** you're eating the perfect number of calories for you, ensuring you lose weight at a healthy rate.

If you wish to be successful, you need to be selling clients the solution to their problem. The way that you achieve the outcome is mostly inconsequential, as far as the client is concerned, provided you get results.

Fly Me Away…

When you're going on holiday, you go on the internet and buy some flights to Barbados. Are you excited about sitting in a giant tin can, zooming over the Atlantic Ocean at 500mph for 12 hours? The person next to you falling asleep on your shoulder? No, probably not…

You *are* excited about laying on the beach, with the golden sand between your toes, crystal clear waves lapping at the shore. A coconut in one hand and a book in the other. That is what you want.

The uncomfortable chair with a fat guy encroaching on your personal space and a child kicking your back for half a day, is the necessary evil to get you there. Unfortunately, they can't teleport you to the other side of the world, yet.

So it is with Personal Training. It is the necessary evil to get the client from fat, sick and unhappy to slim, healthy and confident. Nobody wants a personal trainer, like nobody wants to sit on that plane. They will do it, because they want what is on the other side. They want to be laying on that beach.

Confusing features and benefits is only the start of the problem with the product of Personal Training.

Not only are we selling the means instead of the outcome, but we don't even sell the means very well. How many of your clients get results just by working out?

In our first book, *'The 30/30 Body Blueprint'*, which is for busy women to get fit and lose weight, we have a 5-pillar method. The pillars are:
- Mindset
- Nutrition
- Exercise
- Lifestyle
- Habits

When talking to clients I will reference this, and ask if they agree that you need all 5 of these things to achieve the outcomes that they desire. They always agree.

Without following a nutrition plan, sorting out their lifestyle, stress; the habits and mindsets – what sort of results will the client get?

Exercise is just one component of transforming your body. You know that the client needs all the other stuff outside of the gym too. So, as a top trainer, who cares about your clients; you package it all up and offer them the advice for diet and lifestyle too.

You're Just an Exercise Monkey

The problem is, they haven't bought that. In their mind, they are buying you standing next to them in the gym, pushing them to work harder. *Some* people take the other stuff seriously, do as you say, and inevitably get great results.

Many don't. Many simply do not value the other stuff. They kid themselves that because they're working out and paying you, that is enough for them to see results. Without ever committing to changing their habits outside of the gym.

You know this isn't going to work. Deep down, they probably know it too. But they feel better because they can kid themselves that they are doing something about it. They can even pass responsibility on to you – they're paying you and still not losing weight – it must be your fault!

When the client buys X amount of training sessions, that is all they think they need to do. This is not going to solve their problem – it is only one component of what they need to do.

Not Convinced Yet?

Let's flip it and look at things from the other side. How much do people pay for a nose job? How about a boob job?

They pay thousands to change one small part of how they look. Getting some new bolt-on boobs isn't making them healthier. It's not giving them more energy. It won't make them live longer. They can't run faster or lift more weight. Their posture isn't better (probably worse).

Imagine if you could change *every* part of their body. Totally reinvent their image. Making them slim, toned, shaped. More attractive, better posture AND healthier on the inside too.

That is what happens when you transform your body! All of this, without any anesthetics, scalpels or any of that fun stuff. Just a bit of commitment to changing some lifestyle habits and a little sweat equity.

So, if people are paying thousands for surgery that changes just one small part of their image – how much would they pay to change it all? In a much safer way, that has many, many more benefits for them?

Personal Trainers are seen as a necessary evil – because people do not know what they need to do to properly transform their body. But you do...

Fitness: Better Than Bolt on Boobs

You know what it takes, you even know how to help someone do it.

Well, that is what you must offer people.

When you do so, they will pay you top money, they will get the results they desire and you will genuinely be able to help all your clients.

When you are selling people the thing that they want and need, you can charge way more money for guaranteeing results. You can even do less work to achieve it. You're now selling an outcome, rather than units of your time.

We know this is a paradigm shift that takes some time to get your head around, but when you are selling outcomes rather than time, people will pay more for it to be quicker and easier.

You don't need to drag out their transformation for as long as possible. Make it shorter, and simpler, and they will pay more!

Think about it like this - I go to a dentist because my tooth is wrecked. It has been causing me pain for years, I've just kind of ignored it and lived with it until now - buried my head in my backside.

Eventually one day the pain becomes too much, "I'm going to have to get this tooth sorted".

I've got a choice; the expert down Harley Street who's got this system where I'm in and out in 15 minutes, it feels pain free, and he's known to be the man for this kind of work.
The treatment costs £400 (that's £1,600 by hourly rate).

Or, I could go with the cheap option. He's got a chair and a drill, but he takes 4 hours to do what seems like a similar job. I might give up half way through, as I've heard it's quite painful, especially when I have to sit through it for so long - I know I've given up on painful things before.

But this backstreet dentist only charged £150 an hour - that sounds cheaper. Even though I end up paying more in the end.

Which will you be happier with?

This is what it's like for a client getting a transformation, versus having a PT for 3 years and never getting anywhere significant.

I know, it seems weird as a Personal Trainer to talk about charging more, for less. We are so conditioned by the 'hourly rate' that we lose touch with what people actually want.

Normal People Want to Transform Their Body in the Quickest and Easiest Way Possible

Don't believe people want quick and easy? Look at how many people follow stupid fad diets and buy products which promise:

'RADICAL WEIGHT LOSS IN JUST 3.2 HOURS, LOSE UP TO 74LBS PER MINUTE OR YOUR MONEY BACK!!!!'.

As much as it might hurt your ego, nobody wants to pay you lots of money to spend time with you. While I'm sure that you are a lovely, sparkling personality...people have other things going on.

They want to get the outcome (a new body) and get on with their life!

So how do we deliver the outcome? What do we offer if we're not selling hours of time training with us?

How to Convince Affluent Clients That Online Training Is Right for Them

Are you unsure of how to get affluent clients signed up for online training?

If you wonder why they would choose to work with you online, instead of working with somebody local in person. Or you're not sure what is going to make them choose to buy online training…

Go to http://theprosperouspt.com/bonus for a short video showing you how to convince affluent clients that online training is right for them.

The New Model of Body Transformation

The future of the fitness industry is results based, high-value transformation packages. Encompassing anything and everything that the client needs, to go from where they are now, to where they want to be.

The funny thing is, the client usually needs much less. To be successful, you need to simplify. This is the exact opposite of what most people assume, and do. They think adding more complexity, more stuff and more 'value' is better.

The more advanced your methods, the more complex your plans are, the better the client's outcomes, right?

Not so much. See, the average client is not at an advanced level. The average client *already knows exactly what they need to do to achieve results.*

Come on, you don't think that anyone is shocked to hear they should stop eating donuts for breakfast if they want to lose weight, do you?

For where the client is typically at, you need to offer simplicity and implementation. There is so much information out there; so many trainers, products, diets, regimes that all purport to help them lose weight. It's overwhelming!

They don't know where to start, so they end up doing nothing. Or they start for 2 weeks, haven't seen the 'INCREDIBLE RESULTZZZ!!!!' promised in the infomercial, and switch to a different plan. Repeat ad-infinitum.

Minimum Effective Dose

To effectively help someone, your single role is to help them implement the things that will take them forwards, in the quickest and simplest way possible. Give them the minimum effective dose.

I'm the guy who 'sold' a £3k transformation plan where the training involved me suggesting she goes into her attic, fishes out her old fitness DVD which had been picking up dust for 3 years, and actually did it for once.

Then again. Then three times. Then four times, and repeat 4 times each week.

You get the point - my job is to help her implement. Not to overwhelm her with information. After all, she had got into this situation by not training once in the last 6 months. She didn't have a problem of doing a workout that's only 75% as effective as another one – she had a problem with doing *anything*.

You just need to help people take one step, then the next, and the next.

I had 4 teeth removed, back as a wee 10-year-old. They knock you out with general anesthetic, then go to work pulling your teeth. After they'd finished, they tried to wake me up for about an hour, but I was out of it.

When they administer anesthetic, they give the minimum effective dose. Imagine if they'd given 10-year-old me an adult sized dose. I'd have slept for 3 days! What would that achieve? My teeth would still have been removed in 30 minutes. Now I am just taking up space on their bed, sleeping. Meaning they can't see the next patient, and I can't get back to running around playing football.

They didn't give me 'more value' by giving me more. They wasted my time and hurt their business. More is not better. The minimum effective dose is always best.

When it comes to giving people the means to transformation, less is usually better. Offer your clients the minimum effective dose. They will have a much easier time implementing it, and see better results. Meanwhile, you have less 'busywork' to do, and can help more people.

Do Less, Earn More

Alright so you've convinced me I need to 'do less' to help clients achieve results, and you say they will pay me more for that. I don't get it; how does this work?

Alright, well first, you need to forget that you work in a gym. You're not selling time in the gym. It is possible to still train clients using this new, outcome based model, but it's also possible not to.

In our opinion, many people get better results if you don't have any time in the gym with them. This is for two reasons.

First, they don't see you as 'the exercise person' if you're never in the gym together. They immediately see you as 'the weight loss person' and take on board everything that you advise, not just the exercise. Suddenly, they will follow your dietary advice and everything else!

Secondly, you want to create transformation. This means they will transcend the need to work with you, because they have genuinely changed. Being in the gym with someone can be something of a crutch.

When they must do it themselves, they become self-reliant and this makes it much more likely to be permanent. Now you are offering more value, by freeing them from needing you for the rest of their life to succeed.

You might be thinking that this is all great, but you got in to fitness because you want to be in the gym. If that's the case, you can still sell high-value transformation packages to people and train them in person. That's not the model we are using, but it is possible and much more effective than the standard PT model.

Another alternative, is to make your bread and butter doing high-value online transformations, and then also coach youth athletes, or a semi-pro sports team if you really wish to be in the gym and working with a higher level of athlete. Or you could donate time to less fortunate groups, who need help, but couldn't usually access or afford it.

It depends on what you want as a person. If you like transforming people's lives; when you see that it is not only possible, but in fact easier done online; you might not feel the need to be in the gym with people any longer.

Following on from this, when we talk to people about working completely online, they often raise a few objections like:

"My clients won't follow my stuff"
"Will they train hard enough without me there pushing them?"
"How do I give clients value?"
"Won't the client perceive the value is low, because they don't see me in person?"

Let's look at each of these points in turn.

---

3 Secrets to Ensuring Your Clients Always Check In & Attend Their Calls

Are you worried about clients not turning up for check-ins or attending calls?

What if they disappear because you're lacking the accountability of seeing someone in person?

You want to make sure your clients are compliant…

Go to http://theprosperouspt.com/bonus to discover 3 secrets to ensuring your clients are compliant and always attend their check-ins and calls.

Perhaps they don't follow what you say when they do see you in person, so why would they do so when you're online? How are they going to pay top money, when they're not even seeing you?

Exercise Monkey, No More…

This comes back to selling the outcome, rather than your time. As a Personal Trainer, the client is buying your time doing exercise with them. As far as they're concerned, they are doing what you say (assuming they turn up for their sessions). They see everything outside of the gym as additional stuff, which is not the core of what they're getting from you. They will pick and choose to follow it or not.

When you are selling the outcome of weight loss, and you're not seeing them in person, they only receive what you give them when you speak. This is the entirety of what they get, and because they are buying weight loss, everything you give them is part of that.

They're much more likely to follow what you say, and also more honest about it. They won't bury their head and pretend it's not important if they find it difficult doing something on their own. They will ask for help and face the situation.

The value is not in your time, nor in your presence stood next to them. The value is solely in the outcome. Remember how important weight loss is to your clients, and how it values alongside other methods of changing their image. It's no contest, the value is huge and when the client looks at it from a results perspective – rather than seeing you as someone who does exercise – they will recognise this huge value.

"Will they train hard enough without me pushing them?"

Do most people need to train hard – really?
Or do they just need to train at all?
Remember that 85% of the population have no gym membership, and 2 out of 3 people who do have a membership never use it anyway.

As trainers, we tend to be in a little bubble, because the gym is the environment that we spend all our time, we do not see the world outside of that.

5% of people go to the gym regularly. Do you think more than 5% of the population want to change their body? Conservatively, it's probably 50% or more.

So, for 95% of that population, do they need to train harder...or do they just need to start training at all?

At this level, it doesn't matter what workout they do. Currently they're doing nothing. Doing anything is going to be progress.

(Following this train of thought: You open the size of your market to the ~50+% of people who are not currently going to the gym, but do want to change their body).

When you are selling Personal Training, the client thinks they are buying exercise. Whether they get results or not, they think they're doing the right thing, because they turn up and train a couple of times per week. They justify it to themselves that they are doing something – even if they're not seeing results.

Likewise, and this took me a long time to admit, but it was true. You justify it to yourself that they're coming and training, at least they're better off than they were before. They're a bit fitter and stronger, even if they haven't ultimately seen the results that they desire. That's a piss poor rationalization for your clients not getting results.

Never Worry About Your Clients Not Training Properly

Do you worry about clients not following your programs properly?

Maybe they won't even do the exercise, because they don't know how?

Go to http://theprosperouspt.com/bonus to discover how to ensure your clients do exactly what you say. Even without you there to watch over them in person.

Results Are All That Count

When you are selling the result, that is the only metric that matters. There is no burying your head in the sand and pretending that going to the gym is sufficient progress. Both parties are totally accountable to the ultimate metric that you are trying to change.

All the value you deliver is in the outcome. Both parties see this and both are accountable to achieving that outcome. This is better for both of you. It's how you can get results with every client.

Technophobe?

The final worry that trainers have about working online is the technology and set-up. If you're not a computer person, it can seem scary to try and work solely on the computer.

Well, Tim is the least tech-savvy person we know, and he manages! Honestly the only thing you need to be able to use is Skype. It's just like using the phone. We've all seen the ads where the 80-year-old granny starts using Skype.

You don't need a fancy website (you don't need any website, to be honest). You don't need complex software and funnels. All you need is Email and Social Media for marketing, and Skype for delivery.

At the end of the book is a section called *'How to Start Today'* where we will explain exactly what you need to do to get set up and start working with clients online. Honestly, it is incredibly easy.

The Business Model for High-End Online Body Transformation Coaching

There's many different business models you can use online. Some of them are good, some of them are not. Let's look at the model that we think is the best, and why.

The business model that we recommend is applicable for everyone. If you have illusions of being the next Body Coach and getting famous online, having millions of followers buying your stuff, let me tell you...the chances are slim.

There's very few people who are going to take off like that. After all, if everyone was famous, nobody would be. This is not a good business model because it has a 99.99% failure rate. Yes, the upside is great, but it's like making it in Hollywood. For every Brad Pitt, there are 10,000 35-year-old waiters and car valets, full of resentment and seething anger.

We have huge respect for the Body Coach and anyone else who is successful. We just don't think it's an easily replicable or sensible business model to rely on.

I heard through the grapevine from one of my celeb clients that he used a PR company 3 years ago, and they quoted me £5,000 a month for their basic package. Let's not pretend this was all down to exploding organically on social media. £60,000 a year on PR wouldn't touch the sides with all the other expenses with this business model.

Quick question: Do you care about your clients getting results? Do you want to ensure that they get results?

If you're wanting to take on hundreds, or thousands of clients in a low-price offer, you simply cannot offer a bespoke service.

Go down the volume route and you basically become an 'Internet Marketer' - which is cool, just be aware of that. You're not 'working with clients'. You're offering a 'cookie-cutter' solution that might work for some people, but probably won't work for many.

So, you're not going to get famous. Should you just have an online training package as a down-sell from Personal Training?

No. That is the worst business model possible! You're doing what you would do in person, but for less money. Why would you want to do that? More importantly, nobody wants to buy that.

You might think it takes less time online than doing sessions in person? Let's say you see a client once per week, and you charge them £50 per session. How long do you think you're going to spend in total, talking to this person, writing their program and responding to emails?

You might think an email only takes 2 minutes, but when someone sends you a list of 10 questions and you want to offer a great service and answer them properly, it's going to take half an hour.

When you add up all the time you spend serving this client, directly and indirectly, and you divide it by what you're getting paid, you will probably be doing more work for less money than you would be in person.

Here's the business model that works:

You are offering a better service than Personal Training. It is much more effective and valuable to the client, because you are selling the outcome, instead of the means. The client will understand this and pay more for this.

What you are delivering, really, is coaching.

Coaching differs from training in several key ways which we will look at in a moment. Before we do, think about this:

How much does a coach cost?

Not sure? I personally know people that sell coaching for £50 an hour – about the same as personal training. I also know people that sell coaching for £250,000 per year. I even know of coaches with an hourly rate of £30,000.

So, yes, there is more value in coaching than in training.

What Does a Coach Do Differently to a Trainer?

A coach will work with the client to change their thought patterns and behaviours. To build confidence in the client's internal motivation and thinking, to create permanent change. Training only works for the duration that you continue to do it. Good coaching will create changes for life.

The main difference is that under a coaching model, everything is driven by the client.

If you've ever read biographies about great leaders who take over flagging companies and change the culture – sky-rocketing them to success (Southwest Airlines is a good example). You'll find that if you want people to do something differently, you should involve the ground level people in the discussion. It must be their discussion. Otherwise they feel like they're just being told what to do, and tend not to do it.

Where a trainer will instruct the client exactly what to do, and shout at them and push to make them work harder. The coach will help the client to discover what they need to do, and how to do it on their own. It is their own idea, they become attached to it and work in alignment with it.

Another reason that coaching has so much more value. You are helping the client to have the understanding, confidence and belief in themselves, to be able to do this on their own, for the rest of their life.

You might think coaching costs a lot of money? How much will it cost to have a Personal Trainer for the next 50 years? A lot more than anyone is charging to get the same outcome from coaching.

Now, there's a big caveat here:

This is not for everyone. You must learn the skills as a coach to be able to use this model. If you can't get results with clients, then you have nothing.

Where a trainer can get away with justifying that the client is working out, so they get some benefit, a coach lives and dies by the outcomes. There is no hiding, if you don't get results, you won't get hired.

Results

If you're ok with getting mediocre results and basically earning a steady, but unspectacular, income, being rent-a-friend who chitty-chats with your clients in the gym, then this is not for you.

The trainer will get results with the people who do what you say. The problem is, you are helpless to influence the people who do not follow what you say. In the coaching model, you are not blindly giving recommendations and passing responsibility over to the client to follow them or not.

The coach looks at the whole picture, determines the single thing that the client needs to do to move forwards, and implements that. What might look like basic and obvious things on the outside still need to be actioned, in order to work. Often, the coach is not saying anything that the person doesn't already know. Ask a random on the street, they could advise you to drink more water and eat less sugar.

Honestly, you're going back to basics a lot of the time. The fact is, the basic stuff must be implemented before you even start to think about advanced things.

Most PT's are way too advanced in their knowledge and plans for the average client. If you're working with bodybuilders or athletes it's different, but the clear majority of normal people just need to do the basics right.

The coach's role is to make it as simple and easy to implement as possible, for the client. Simplicity comes after complexity. The coach will have all the knowledge, information and experience, to pick the single, simplest, most effective thing for the client to implement, which moves them forwards to the greatest degree.

It's probably not anything the client doesn't already know. The simple fact is, the knowledge is doing them absolutely no good what so ever, until they implement it in to action. You must recognise that results come from action. Check your ego and help people do the most basic next step possible.

You don't need to impress clients with knowledge; you need to inspire them to act. That is what the coach does.

When it comes to speaking to a potential client, they likely do not know what a Body Transformation Coach does. You have appealed to them by speaking on their level about their problems and desires. They don't know what you actually do to achieve the outcomes that you achieve with your clients.

You need to learn how to frame yourself as the high-value answer to their problem. To explain what you do and why they need your help. This is very different to selling Personal Training. The positioning is all different, and to be successful, you're going to have to look at things in a totally different perspective.

We go in to marketing and selling coaching in later chapters. First, let's look at what we are selling. What does a coaching package look like?

Coming up we will expand on the business model and what goes in to a coaching package. This is what we recommend. We recommend it because it is what we do and it is what we coach other people to do. It works. It has been replicated by dozens of people, with hundreds of clients in all sorts of different places.

Before that, we're going to give you a quick rundown on how to coach your clients, and some important mindsets towards your business.

How to 'Hynotise' Clients to Ensure They Follow Everything You Say

Are you worried that clients will not be compliant?

Perhaps you think they will lie to you about how well they have been sticking to the plan?

Maybe you're worried that without the accountability of seeing them, they are going to be less likely to follow your advice? After all, many of your in-person clients now don't always follow your advice outside of the gym, right?

Go to http://theprosperouspt.com/bonus to discover how to 'hypnotise' clients, to ensure they follow everything you say.

3 HOW TO DELIVER HIGH-VALUE ONLINE COACHING

A sticking point for a lot of trainers who want to deliver online coaching, and maybe even feel confident in marketing and selling it, is that they do not know how to deliver the coaching to a client once they have them.

Obviously teaching you everything there is to know about coaching is beyond the scope of this book. Something Tim covers in his mentorship is exactly what he does with clients to get transformational results that are better than in-person training. Here we're going to go over some basics, to give you enough information to get started and see some success.

Like with your own clients, telling you everything about everything is not going to be productive. It is overwhelming and cannot be actioned. Anyway, the first and most important thing to cover is this:

Getting the Client to Do the Work

You cannot do it for them. They must be responsible for implementing things.

They are the ones doing the workouts, eating the meals, drinking the water, sleeping at night and all the other things we know they need to do to achieve results.

Personal Trainers typically have their clients doing exceptionally well in the workout part of that equation – obviously – but leave it completely up to chance on everything else.

Sure, you give advice; telling them how to eat, etc. but whether or not they follow it is pretty random. You know clients get great results when they do follow it, but some people just won't, for whatever reason.

A successful coaching relationship empowers the client to take responsibility and action on their own. Not helplessly passing all responsibility onto you.

Expectations

This starts by setting the right expectation and creating boundaries. When you communicate from the start that the client can get results on their own, which they will be able to sustain forever, because they develop the thinking patterns to make decisions on their own – they will be on board with that.

> *"Can you see that it is most beneficial for your results that you can do this yourself in the years to come?*
>
> *That you can make decisions – the right decisions – on your own, given the right framework?*
>
> *I assume you don't want to still be working with me in 2… 5… 20-years-time? But you do want to maintain success in this area of your life?"*

Of course, they will want that. It's important that you have this conversation early, so that everything you do together is framed in this context.

Boundaries

The next step is to set boundaries. You're there to help your clients when they need it, but you are not there to babysit them 24/7. They need to be able to make basic decisions themselves. They need to build confidence and belief that they can achieve this on their own.

Honestly, that is often the biggest reason they have not seen success in this part of their life before. Most regimes work if they are followed. Most people have seen successful weight loss results for a few weeks, before 'falling off the wagon'.

They simply don't have the self-belief to maintain it. There is no magic formula that is a well-hidden secret. The general public know enough to apply the 80-20 rule to their fitness and be successful. They just don't do it, because they don't believe in themselves. They don't believe it can be so simple.

Setting boundaries means telling them when you will help them, and when you won't. Then sticking to that.

Clients will initially try to push the boundaries, that is completely natural. It's human nature to push boundaries and see what we can get away with. It is integral to their success that you remain rigid in your boundaries. Do not get sucked in to letting your boundaries down.

Here is what we mean:

You've told a client that you will speak with them once per week, and they have agreed to personal responsibility. That they should work things out for themselves, within the framework you have given, and act on that.

They can check in on your scheduled check-ins, but they do not need to ask you every little detail. They should use their best judgement. This will build their confidence and belief.

They've agreed to this, and you have given them a basic plan to implement. However, they are now hitting you up, desperately 'needing' to know if it is better for them to eat blueberries or raspberries as a snack. Something that in the grand scheme of things honestly does not matter one iota.

The temptation for you is to answer them. To just tell them that it doesn't matter, or whatever you would say.

You cannot do this. You cannot indulge them.

You must maintain your boundary and let them think about it themselves. If you don't respond to them, they will figure it out and decide for themselves.

This probably seems like a very minor thing to you right now, but it is about maintaining the boundary. Setting the precedent that they can decide on their own.

Can you see how, if they cannot make this simple decision on their own, they stand little chance of being able to find resolutions to bigger problems.

You must get them used to thinking for themselves. Building their 'decision muscle' and taking responsibility.

I asked my client Bunmi to use My Fitness Pal in the first week. We spoke on Monday, and I asked her to start using it on Tuesday (the next day). Here's what she told me:

She said, "*I used My Fitness Pal and it was great. I went to work the next day and tried to choose food in the canteen that gave me a decent meal, and left me enough calories for later.*

Whatever I chose, everything just took me way over my calories. I was ok that day, I did what I could, but what I realized was that I needed to do something different tomorrow.

There's no way I could fit in my calories like this. So, the next day I went to buy my lunch from the supermarket down the road, because I knew I could easily fit within my calories that way".

If I'd not taught her how to make decisions, and built her confidence, she would have wasted 6 days not knowing what to do. Instead she just got on with it and didn't even need to ask me.

She had good lunches that she enjoyed, felt full and easily stayed within her calories. She solved that problem herself. From then on, whenever challenges came up, she was empowered to make decisions and act on them herself.

If she isn't able to figure that small thing out, how would she ever be able to figure this whole weight loss thing out for the rest of her life?

You want clients who are empowered to find resolutions to problems – not clients who are coming to you with every minor problem possible.

That is the opposite of being self-reliant. That is being completely reliant on you to babysit them. Unfortunately, you cannot be with them 24 hours a day and they are going to be left stranded on their own, feeling helpless to make the right decision without you.

As you can imagine, people will usually revert to the wrong decision in that situation.

It might seem initially like it doesn't matter, or that you're not serving your client by refusing to indulge their need for help. You must stay strong and do it. It's in their best interests for them to be able to make decisions alone.

Remember that you have already framed how this relationship works at the start. You can simply turn it back on them. Say;

> *"Remember you told me that you want to become self-reliant and not need me for every little decision, right?*
>
> *Can you see that you making a decision and taking action on your own is more important – in the long run – than any negligible difference between eating blueberries or raspberries?"*

They're not stupid. They will agree with what you are doing when you frame it in this way.

You'll be surprised how often you get another message half an hour later telling you that they worked it out for themselves. They will often thank you for making them think for themselves. They know that this is how they will learn.

Getting Dressed for Your First Date

We tend to blow up a decision or minor problem as being the most important thing in the world when it is at the forefront of our mind. Every little thing becomes life or death. You know how crippling it is trying to decide what to wear for a first date you've been looking forward to, right?

When we take a step back, we can see that it isn't that important. We are 'majoring in the minor'. Yet in the moment, we don't feel like that.

You simply have to pull your client away from the situation from time to time, allowing them to see the bigger picture – rather than being stuck inside it. They will thank you.

"Just post on Facebook…"

When I first hired – and paid a lot of money – to my business mentor he told me to do 2 things in the first week. To set my income targets and make some posts on Facebook. That was all. I'm left wondering why I have paid so much money for someone to tell me to set goals and post on Facebook.

Of course, I already know I should have goals and be posting on Facebook – what am I paying for?

Of course, I also wasn't doing those 2 things. Within 5 days I had a new £6k (in-person) client that had come from a Facebook post.

That was when it clicked for me and I saw the value of *implementing* something basic. His skill as a coach wasn't – in this instance – in the depth of his knowledge, but in his ability to get me to action the very basics.

Creating Breakthroughs

Now that you have boundaries, you need to create change in your client's daily actions. This is where most trainers overwhelm their clients with complicated diet plans and far more information than they can put to action in one go.

In the first week of working with a new client, we will have our coaching call and discuss several things. How they got where they are now, what their goals are, what their potential struggles are going to be. At the end of the call, our take away advice will typically look something like this:

> *"Drink 2+ liters of water per day. Get a big bottle and carry it around. Make sure it is empty by the time you go to bed.*
>
> *Do some form of exercise 3x per week. Anything you wish – it could be walking around the block".*

That's all.

It's like my mentor with the Facebook thing. We *could* give them lots of complicated, advanced information – but why?

Take the low hanging fruit. If they're chronically dehydrated, fixing that is going to move the needle more than anything else.

It's what we call a big rock.

You know the analogy of filling a bucket, right? Big rocks first, then smaller rocks slip between the cracks and finally sand will slip between the smaller rocks.

To get the most volume in the bucket, you have to start with the big rocks first. If you put the sand in first, nothing else will fit.

The big rocks in fitness are the things that have the greatest impact for the least effort – like drinking more water.

The biggest struggle with this is entirely a mental one on your part. You feeling like you need to 'give more value'.

If you believe that value is in information, that would be valid.

However, when you are coaching, the value is not in information. The value is in results. Results come from *implementation.* Telling someone to do something very basic like drinking water is the most valuable thing you can offer them, because *when they actually do it,* they see the biggest positive outcome.

Telling them about nutrient timing and macro's is useless. They're not going to be able to implement it. You should build momentum over time to get to the more complex stuff. Besides, they'd still be chronically dehydrated, even if they did manage to follow your macro's.

Give them big rocks first – like drinking water, fixing breakfast and doing some form of movement.

Momentum

Is walking around the block the most effective way to train? No, of course not.

However, if this person hasn't worked out for 6 months, it is manageable for them. They can do it and start to build that all important momentum. In a few weeks, they will be doing the workouts you think are most effective, but right now, they need to start with the workout they can actually do.

Small wins and momentum lead to big wins and more momentum. Steep obstacles lead to failure, loss of confidence and belief, and inevitably giving up.

You have to get your client moving along the behaviour continuum from where they are now, to fulfilling all the behaviours they need to fulfill, to have the body they want.

We need to have empathy with our clients. As trainers, we are typically so far away from the average person who doesn't like exercise, hasn't a clue what to do, or any confidence in themselves physically.

Knowing the 'right' thing, the *best* workout, the latest, most cutting edge techniques is not what clients need. Clients will get excited and say they can do these complicated workouts, but in reality, they can't. The level they are at is much lower than you imagine. You should consciously start at the beginning and meet them where they are, not where they wish / kid themselves they are.

Trying to jump straight to the end is simply not going to work. That is what most people do when they join the gym and start a hardcore diet, follow it for 2 weeks and see good results…

Then stop and immediately go back to where they started. It was unsustainable because it was far too far away from their current behaviours to be maintained.

For an example of a full weekly breakdown go to http://theprosperouspt.com/bonus.

Remember, the value in your service comes from the results you get for your clients. Not the amount of knowledge or complexity your programs display. The simplest option is usually the best.

4 YOUR MINDSET: HOW YOU MUST APPROACH COACHING

Think about where you're at in your business right now.

You're probably doing ok, right? You're getting by. It's comfortable enough.

You work long hours and don't make as much as you might wish, but you're not going to go hungry any time soon, you know. It's not so bad?

Let's extend that out over 5 or 10 years...

Would you still be happy?

If you've not progressed over the last decade? Maybe you put your prices up by £5 a couple of times, but that was just in keeping with inflation and rising gym rents.

Working all the hours under the sun is cool when you're young. It's kind of a rite of passage to building a successful business or career. What happens later though? When you want to settle down and get married? What about when you have kids? Do you still want to be leaving the house at 5am and returning at 9pm? Missing most of your kids' lives?

At this stage, you're going to be in a corner. Weddings and kids are expensive. Plus, you'll probably have bought a house and got a hefty mortgage to pay. Now you have no choice *but* to work as much as possible. You need all the money you can get your hands on to pay the ever-mounting bills.

Does this sound like where you want to be? Are you going to be doing this from now until you retire?

I'm sure most of us never imagined that. In any field, as you become experienced and get to the top of the game, you generally attain more income, more freedom, more power and more control.

Well, if you keep using the old Personal Training model you get none of that. All that you get, is more hours in the gym.

(AKA less time with your family and kids, less free time or holidays).

This is important to think about, because the actions that you take now set the tone for where you will be in 1, 5, 10 years' time.

Do you think you would be happy if your life is the same in 5 years' time?

It's going to take a shift to change that. Doing more/better of what you're already doing is not it. That just creates more problems, further diminishing your free time and freedom to build a real business.

You might be self-employed, but right now you essentially have a job. You turn up at the office (gym), punch your time clock in, put in the hours and at the end of the day, punch out.

Ok, you don't have a boss – though some of your clients are probably just as bad. Remember, you don't have a steady pay check, benefits, holidays or a pension either.

To attain the kind of freedom and income you desire. That allows you to live comfortably, have the time to see your kids grow up, take a few weeks holiday each year and pay the mortgage without worry, you need a *business*.

A business has scale; it can grow beyond the limited hours of manual labour you can put in to it. It can grow in income, without you having to create more hours in the day to give away.

It can be run without you being tied to a specific location; like being in the gym every morning at 5am.

The business owner (you) is actually in control of the business, the income and the time. Right now, your clients are in control and you're just spinning plates to try and keep them all happy.

Case Study: Karolina

When Karolina came in, she was charging decent money for 1-1 PT in central London. It looked great on the surface, but she had no way of getting new clients. Very fearful because some of her clients paid a lot of money, so she bent over backwards for them. They would sometimes take advantage, but she couldn't have the conversations she needed to, due to worrying that they might leave.

She really wanted to be more than a trainer, a coach. Coming on board, Karolina struggled initially, getting knocked back quite a lot. She just wasn't able to get clients signed up.

She wanted freedom to move out of London. Feeling very frustrated with herself, knowing she has a really good product, but not able to find a way to get it out to people. Clients get great results, but reaching new people was a struggle.

On December 1st (when most fit-pros make no money) she made her first sale, and from there it clicked. It was an easy sale, and another one followed the next day. Then another a week after. December was by far her best ever month in business, making £8.5k.

"What Does It Take to Build a Real Business?"

The lifeblood of any business is sales. Without selling, the business is nothing. Without selling, you cannot help any clients. Without selling, you cannot grow and expand. Without selling, you cannot sustain the business.

Transformation Happens in The Sale

Let us remind you of our personal story.

We were business partners for many years in London when we were both still Personal Trainers and were looking for a way to create a scalable business. We both had our goals which we knew Personal Training was not going to allow us to attain.

Phil wanted to travel the world and be able to work remotely from anywhere. Tim wanted a high income that allowed him to buy a house and work from home, to start a young family.

For 3 years, we were working on a business and everyone around us thought we were being successful. We were achieving a lot. We were running a bootcamp company with the intention of franchising it to other Personal Trainers. Stepping back from delivering sessions, to grow the company and manage the other trainers. We had:

- Written and published a best-selling book
- A beautiful, interactive, unique website
- Professional videos telling our story
- Appeared in dozens of national and international newspapers and magazines
- Trained celebrities
- Had bootcamps in up to 6 locations at once in London
- Taken on people to run the bootcamps for us
- Started the first franchise

Now, here is what we never did:

- Made any real money

The truth is, we were financing the whole operation from the money we made Personal Training. The business was consistently losing money.

Phil even started scaling down his PT hours to free more time working on the business, leading him in to a financial hole, because the business wasn't paying out. It continued consuming more money, and after taking the risk of dropping hours, he wasn't making enough from PT to get by for very long.

It was a race against time that we lost. Now it is incredibly obvious that we were always going to fail, and here is why...

We Weren't Selling!

It's not that we feared selling. When someone did come for a trial session at a bootcamp, or when we wanted to find a franchisee to come on board, sales were closed with ease. Problem was, we were always deferring the act of getting clients.

We did everything to build our brand, position ourselves in the market. Obsessed over the image that came across in our videos. Re-wrote our website dozens of times.

The problem was, none of this led to us getting clients. All the marketing we were doing was useless.

We did things like:

- Brand building on social media (instead of client getting)
- Press and publicity

...and it brought us absolutely nothing.

We did some things right, we got some clients through SEO and being top of Google rankings, but that was passive. We had to just sit and wait for the trickle of people to find us when they were searching. We got maybe a couple of good leads per month like this.

We were also E-mailing our list, which is where most of our clients came from. We got this half-right, but the problem was still the offer. We were not offering the right thing to our potential clients, so they were not buying at the level we needed them to.

We literally spent years doing all of these things that we thought were marketing – but deferring a return on the effort and investment for the future. Our favourite sentence was;
"After X happens, it will really take off".

After our website is finished. After we start ranking in SEO. After we get a new video on our homepage. After we publish our book. After we are in this newspaper.

Of course, nothing significant ever happened after any of these events we were so sure were going to 'make us'.

We spent a lot of money, weeks of preparation, and hours practicing our speech in advance of our book launch. We had a bunch of celebrities there, a load of journalists and all our clients. It was a good night, again it was stroking our egos, making us feel big time. Yet when the dust settled it made absolutely no difference in our business.

We got a little bit of coverage, that brought no clients in. Back to square one and the book launch party was a big net loss.

Does this sound familiar?

Probably. It is what most Personal Trainers go through. More than that, it is what most small businesses go through.

That is how we ended up in that situation. We did all the courses, read all the books and followed all the marketing tribe-building gurus, but nobody ever told us to go out and start selling!

You get away with it in Personal Training, because clients bring recurring income. You don't need many clients, and each one tends to pay you a decent amount of money, every month, for a long time. Once you're on your feet and established, you only need a couple of new clients per year.

We had bigger aspirations and were trying to aggressively grow our bootcamps, which meant we needed hundreds of clients. It simply wasn't going to happen in the passive trickle that most small businesses get new clients.

It literally astounds me now that we spent so much money on some things. We were paying £1,500 for PR - PER MONTH - for about 6 months. We spent about £3,000 on professional videos for our website that had about 100 views – total!
Now that we have seen the light and figured out what it means to market and sell, if you give either of us a £1,500 per month marketing budget we will 10x that money in about a week.

How?

(and this is what you are going to need to do to grow your business)

Direct-response marketing and selling. More on that later.

We're going to get in to how to do this later in the book. For now, we are just looking at the mindset of business. As you can see from our failures, without marketing and selling, you don't have a business. You have a time and money black hole that unapologetically consumes *everything*.

More Mindset Shifts…

Something you must realise about sales…

We both thought we could sell. On the rare occasion that a potential client would stumble across our website or find us somehow, we had a great rate of closing sales. Likewise, when someone took up a free trial PT session, we almost always got them as a client. We thought we could sell...

Problem is, that is not selling.

When someone is coming to you, and they're already ready to buy what you offer, you are not selling. You're taking an order.

We call this 'not sticking your foot in your mouth' selling.

Literally, all you need to do, is avoid doing anything so stupid that you scare off the dead-cert client.

While a lot of trainers still manage to mess this up, because they're so uncomfortable asking for money, the majority can close these sales.

Tim will recount the story of how he figured out that, really, he didn't know how to sell.

After we finally let go of that previous business (which we should have done a year before we did, but that's another story), I hired a business coach to sort my shit out.
Although that business had failed, I was still making steady income from Personal Training. I had a couple of very high value clients and was comfortable, without having to work so many hours that I had no free time, to work on growing my business.

That wasn't what I wanted though. I had much bigger aspirations and I finally took the plunge and invested £5,000 in a business coach. I'd thought about doing it 6 months earlier, but didn't commit to it.

This time something had changed and I was really serious. Time to put my money where my mouth was.

Anyway, one of the first things he did was challenged me on my ability to sell. Now there was a mindset shift.

I could sell to people who were ready to buy what I was selling (not sticking my foot in my mouth), but I'd never sold to someone who wasn't sure.

Even though I was charging top money for PT, I had managed to find some hyper-wealthy people for whom it was pocket change. I'd never got a normal person to commit to a transformation that was a financial stretch. I'd never sold to anyone for whom it was a risk to commit.

What I wanted to do, was sell online coaching and sell it at top money.

There's a big difference between online coaching and Personal Training, as discussed earlier. People will go looking for a Personal Trainer, because they think it is the answer to their problem. Nobody is looking to hire an online coach, because they're not aware that it is a solution for them.

That means you must position yourself and present your value to someone who is not already looking to buy from you.

Of course, *you are the perfect solution* for them. Don't get disheartened.

The only problem is, they're not aware of that, until you give a compelling reason for them to believe it. You're ahead of the market. Online coaching hasn't trickled down to the awareness of the masses yet. Educating prospects on why you are a better option than a Personal Trainer, is selling.

Selling is convincing someone to take an action that they were not previously committed to taking.

Ethical selling is convincing someone to take an action *that is the right course of action for them*, that they were not previously committed to taking.

If you offer the best solution to someone's serious problems, it is your moral and ethical duty to sell to them. If you genuinely help people to better their lives and overcome a true problem, then selling to them is the only right course of action. Not selling is doing them a complete disservice.

More on this in the sales section.

To take someone from unaware of what you do, or why they need your help, to paying you a significant amount of money, which can be uncomfortable for them – this, is selling.

Continuing down the mindset theme. You have to be comfortable taking people on this journey and making them an offer to help them, assuming it is the right fit for them. If it's not, they won't buy anyway, but you shouldn't even pitch them. Pass them on to someone better suited to help them.

Doing this, you are going to encounter a lot of rejections. A lot of people are not going to commit, for a variety of reasons.

As you get better at selling, this will happen less, and as you gain experience, you are better able to qualify who are the right people to be speaking to in the first place.

Still, you will get told "no" more often than people buy, and you need to be OK with this.

If you define yourself, your worth, by what the latest person you spoke to opted to do; you're not going to be very happy. People are going to reject you. It just means they're not ready, or the problem is not large enough, for them to pay top money to fix it.

You can't let it alter your belief in yourself, this would negatively impact your other clients, who have chosen to invest with you. It does take time and the more money you're making, the less you grow to care about a rejection. That said, it is something that you should address.
You need to develop an abundance mindset; where you know that if one client says "no", there is always another right around the corner who will say "yes". Every "no" is a step closer to the next "yes". You want to help this person, but you're not affected by the outcome. If they say no, that is OK.
This starts as a mental exercise, you should tell it to yourself, and it will develop in to your natural thought patterns, as you see greater success.

Finding Your Perfect Client

Who would be your perfect client? There's many factors to this:
- the type of person who you get along with and enjoy helping
- the person who really needs your help
- the person who you are best positioned to help
- the person who values what you do highly
- the person in the most pain/most need of help
- the person for who you will make the biggest impact

These are all factors to consider when looking at your 'perfect client'.

Where to Find Affluent Clients, Who Will Pay £2k For an Online Body Transformation

Are you on board with the idea, but wondering where to find clients who will pay £2k for an online body transformation?

Go to http://theprosperouspt.com/bonus to discover exactly where to find these clients.

This person does not have to be hugely wealthy. It just needs to be important enough for them to pay for it. Would you be surprised if I told you that over the last year I have worked with a client whose yearly income was £22,000 and another who earned £23,000? What about one who makes just £13,000?

That's not a lot of money to then spend £2,000 on a body transformation, is it?
The fact is, you do not need to be meeting super rich business moguls and oil barons to charge top money for your services.

What you do need to do, is to deliver huge value and be able to clearly articulate that to your client. The fact is, there are (lots of) people out there in enough pain to pay £2,000 and much more to get their body sorted.

Honestly, the average Personal Training client spends much more than that over their lifetime. The only difference is, you are getting the money up front and delivering the result in a short time-frame. Instead of dragging out the time it takes them to achieve their goals – as though this somehow delivers them more 'value'!

Remember: people do not care to pay for spending time with you, they want to achieve an outcome and will pay to do so quickly and efficiently.

One of the most interesting things that we have learnt and now want to get across to you, is this:

The Price You Charge Is Where the Market Will Meet You

What we mean is this...

If you are valuing your service at £30 per hour, you are going to find clients who value what you do at £30 per hour.

If you are valuing your service at £2,000, you are going to find clients who value what you do at £2,000.

Now who do you think is going to be a better client – someone who values changing their body at £30 or at £2,000?

Pricing is not determined by what anyone else in the market is doing. You are separating yourself from Personal Trainers and offering a completely different service.

Pricing is determined by how much value the client places on the outcome. Many people will happily pay £2,000 to change their body – as we discussed earlier – and these are the people who you want to be working with.

Alright, so we're on board so far.
"Where are we going to find these people though? Everyone in my area/my network/my email list is a price shopper who wants to pay £30".

Here's the deal. If I decide I want to go fishing, I grab a piece of stale bread, attach it to a piece of string and plonk it in the nearest puddle of water – do I expect to catch anything?

Doubtful.

If I want to catch deep sea fish, I'm going to need a big boat, one of those reinforced rods, someone to take me out on to the ocean, etc.

If I'm after salmon, I need to go to a fresh water river, have the full-body waterproof get up and fly fishing line, right?

You need to have the right equipment and be in the right place, to catch the fish that you're looking for.

First, you need to decide what type of fish you want, then you need to go to where they are.

Define your perfect client, then go and find them where they are. The beauty of working online is that there are NO restrictions on who you can work with. They don't need to be in your geographic area, or able to get to your gym. You've opened the floor to anybody in the world.

If you want to work with high-flying corporate executives, you can. Regardless of where they are, or where you are.

How to Choose Your Niche Market

Here's how to choose your niche market – the subset of people that you serve.

Niche Market

A niche market is a specific subset of the market that you choose to serve.

We choose to work in a niche because it means our marketing is more relevant and specific to the people we are trying to serve. Our service is more aligned with their specific goals and the problems that they need to overcome. Rather than trying to be a generalist and serve everybody.

Examples of a niche market you can work with include:
Brides
Post-divorce professional women in their 30's
Male entrepreneurs making £100-500k

Look at what you have experience in and empathy with. Look at who you've most enjoyed working with, and got great results with before. Look at where your passions lie, and who you would love to help for free, if you could. These are a good place to start thinking, but you also need your niche to be economically viable.

There's a few criteria that make a niche a good choice, from a business perspective. Primarily, there needs to be a high level of pain that you can solve.

Pain…Is Good

People are more strongly motivated by moving away from pain than they are by moving towards pleasure. For someone to come on board, pay you well, take it seriously and achieve incredible results; there needs to be something driving them. Something that makes this important enough for them to pay to get it fixed, urgently.

You might need to help them discover this pain sometimes, but that's all part of the process.

I was on a call recently with a lady, and I asked her how important it was to transform her body, on a scale of 1-10. She replied that it was a 5.

> *"OK, do you know what your BMI is, by any chance?"*

She didn't, so I asked if it was OK to work it out. We did, and it came out at 38.

> *"Tell me what you know about the BMI categories?"*

She listed the categories and mentioned the top category as 'obese' – I asked what category she thinks she is in, with a BMI of 38.

"I think I'd be clinically obese"

> *"OK, tell me, what do you know about the health complications of people in this category?"*

She went on to start listing heart disease, cancer, etc.

When she'd finished, I chose to look deeper in to diabetes. I think talking about heart disease and cancer is a bit too morbid, but diabetes is a good place to meet them.

> *"Did you know that when you have diabetes, it doesn't go away. You have it forever?"*

She kinda knew that.

> *"...and that you will have to take injections every day, for the rest of your life. It's not something you can wait until it happens and then do something about it. It's too late then."*

Ok, she didn't know that...

> *"Would it surprise you to know that your feet can fall off, you can go blind"*

She murmured in agreement.

> *"Do you know how much more likely you are to get diabetes if you are in the obese category, versus the overweight category?"*

She wasn't sure...

> *"You're 18 times more likely to get diabetes."*

Silence for a few seconds...

You could feel the tension through the phone.

"Oh."

> *"I know you said this is a 5/10 a moment ago, but help me out here, what are your thoughts on this now?"*

Suddenly, she's a 10 out of 10 and says she NEEDS to do something about this, immediately.

Now, this was just exploring 1 thing, out of the many, many reasons she might want to lose weight.

It might seem like this is not a very nice thing to do to people, but the fact is it's 100% true. Everything that I told her was a fact.

I'd much rather make someone feel uncomfortable now, and hopefully kick them in to making a change (with me or through other means) than have her feet fall off in a few years' time when she does have diabetes.

You're doing the client a service by helping them see how important this is. Not letting them pretend that it's OK and bury their head in the sand.

Of course, you need the knowledge and the skills to do this in the right way, for them to come to their own conclusions about it.

If you just tell someone, they will become defensive and reject it; and you. To present something in a way that people are going to believe, you have to allow them to think of it themselves. You're doing people a great service when you help them to see how important this is for them – you could be saving their life.

Now, do you think this lady values transforming her body and long term health at £2,000 or more – regardless of whether or not she is wealthy?

Return on Investment

The more easily your niche can see a direct return on their investment, the easier it will be for them to see the huge value in your service. Going back to the lady above, would you pay £2,000 to save your feet from falling off?

If you work with business people and executives; people who have been solely focused on their work; to the detriment of their health and everything else. They're starting to break down. Their health is deteriorating; energy levels are tanking. Suddenly, they can't focus or get anything done.

They fear getting sick and not being able to work. They will lose money and everything that they have worked so hard for. Stressed, overworked and worried that they can't go on.

In just a month of working with you, they are going to see a very direct return on their investment. They will make more money in their business. It's a really easy sell when it is this obvious how much they will benefit.

Of course, not everyone will see monetary return on investment. It might be health, confidence, relationship, social, self-worth. These are all still extremely important to people.

Your perfect client will see a large return on their investment. They *need* to do this.

"But What If...?"

Let's address some of the reasons people have for not honing in on one niche.

First of all, many are concerned about not having enough clients. In person this *may* be an issue; people will only travel so far and your total audience is in the thousands or 10's of thousands in your immediate area.

Charles Poliquin says that generally people will only travel 15 minutes to go to the gym. Of course, some people will travel longer, but most people won't. Even the ones that do, the travel time can begin to come a problem and they're more likely to leave sooner.

Online your audience is literally the whole world. 7 billion people. No matter how targeted your niche is, there will be more than enough people for you to work with.

One of the guys in my mentorship works with single City/Wall Street guys in their late 30's who have just come out of a relationship. This is a very tight niche, but there's plenty enough of them to build a solid business there.

You can become the go-to person in that niche and really become relevant to the right people. Yes, you will turn off some people who are not right for you, but you attract the people that are right for you.

One of the niches we were involved in was the bridal niche. Training women for their wedding day. Whenever we went to events and spoke to people, they were immediately interested in what we did.

"Oh my friend/sister/co-worker is getting married, I'll introduce you."

How often do people say that, when you say you are a Personal Trainer?

"Oh my friend/sister/co-worker is fat, I'll introduce you." - Yeh right.

People generally roll their eyes - "oh, another Personal Trainer. Boring".

Maybe they will hit you up for some free advice that they're not going to follow.

When you're in a niche market, everyone knows what you do and who you help. It gives clarity and makes you stand out from the millions of other people who all do the same thing.

People immediately respond positively, because it's something they have probably not heard before. Whereas everyone knows 5 Personal Trainers, and it is absolutely nothing noteworthy whatsoever.

What about if you lose out on people who might want to work with you, because they don't fit your niche?

Really, do you want to work with anyone who has a wallet and a pulse? This is a scarcity mindset that comes from Personal Training, because you're constantly in a dog fight with all your competitors. You will take any business that you can get.
In that unstructured, insecure and broken model, it is built on scarcity and it is completely normal. In the new model, there is no need to work with anyone who is not a perfect fit for you. There's an abundance of people out there, and now you have access to all of them.

Focus on finding the right people for you – not anyone who is willing to pay you.

Your business will be much more enjoyable; clients will be low maintenance and fun to work with. They will get incredible results; you will be fulfilled and they will be over the moon.

Your Perfect Client Avatar

When you have decided upon a niche, you can create your perfect client avatar. This is the demographics and characteristics of your perfect client.

Client Avatar

A client avatar is the image that you create of your 'perfect client'.

It takes the information you have about your niche market and humanises it. Making your client avatar the 'profile' of your perfect client. You use the client avatar to guide how you communicate with your market.

Often you are not in your own target market, by having a client avatar you can get into the head of your prospects and empathise with how they are thinking and feeling.

The first level of a client avatar is basic demographic information, but the second level is where it really becomes important. You build up a picture of your avatar's fears and desires, this is what will drive them to act and change their body.

When you understand this on a deep level you can communicate with your market in their own language and they feel that you genuinely understand and care about them.

The need to tie down your avatar is important, because that is who you will be marketing to. It's very hard to get any traction when you just throw generic stuff out in to the world, hoping to attract everyone. They will simply respond with a "so what?".

There's nothing that separates you from anyone else or particularly speaks to that client. It is arrogant and misguided to expect them to somehow know that you are the best, or in any way different to anyone else.

When you speak directly to your avatar, you are calling out problems and characteristics that sound exactly like them. You will often get the response of "It's like you're inside my head, talking to me".

Which do you think is a stronger selling message?

Now, you're never going to find someone who exactly fits your avatar down to every single detail. You're looking for similar groups of people, with similar characteristics, who will respond to your messaging.

If someone has taken the step to get in touch, something you said has obviously spoken to them, so they're probably going to be a fit.

Don't use trying to find your 'perfect avatar' as an excuse to not have sales conversations and make offers to people. If they're seeking you out to help them, it is because they believe that you have the answers that they're looking for.

Perhaps you think your perfect client will be in their 30's, but this person is 43. That's OK – you can still help them.

The point of the avatar isn't that it needs to be an exact match. It's the general story that you are telling. If they respond to it, you are matching up. The problems, situation, goals are what count. The demographics and avatar are just making it more likely you are going to find those people.

They make the abstract in to something more quantifiable, that you can use to find the right clients. It's important to remember that to grow your business, you need to be selling.
If someone wants to talk to you about helping them, they are probably going to be the right fit for your business. Especially if your messaging is targeted to a niche.

Will you not get bored working with the same kind of people all the time?

While you want your clients to all roughly fit your avatar, there is still going to be massive variability. Everyone is a unique person, with different personalities, situations, life experiences, etc.

You are helping them all move toward similar goals, but the day-to-day of what it takes to get there will differ vastly.

For example, this book is written to help Personal Trainers to earn more money and have more freedom, with online coaching. Think about you and the other guys in your gym. I'd be willing to bet that everyone wants more money and freedom. You're probably all around similar ages. Basically, you all fit the same avatar.

Are you all the same? Do you have the same struggles? Are your goals and reasons for wanting it all the same? Are your strengths and weaknesses the same?

Of course, they're not, right? You're all different. Working with each of you would be different. You all fit the same avatar though.

How to Get Your First High-Value Online Client Without Even Needing a Website or Complicated Funnel

Awesome work if you're ready to get started right away…

But what if you don't have a website, or any online funnel set up to get clients?

Go to http://theprosperouspt.com/bonus to discover how to get your first high-value online client, without a website or complicated funnel.

Why You Don't Need Fame or a Big Profile

You see the biggest names in the industry; millions of Instagram followers and Facebook fans, best-selling books and a large audience. It's natural to rationalize that they are successful because of their reach and fame. To become successful like them, and earn that much money, you need to be on the TV too, right?

Nope. You really don't.

Case Study: Adam

When Adam first joined the mastermind, he was expecting his first child in 3 months' time. He had realised now that he needed to do something before his kid arrives. There was little choice, he just wasn't making enough money to provide the kind of life he wanted for his young family.

He considered leaving the industry, to do something else. He's a great coach, gets great results, but he knew he needed to do something different. He would do what it took to provide for his family in the way that he wanted to. He wasn't scared to back himself and invest in the right help to reach his goals.

He had always wanted to be online. He's fully online now, because he didn't want to live in the UK at the time. When he came on board, he pushed himself, straight into selling a £2k program. Within 4 months, he had his first £10k month. Within 6 months his first 15k month. Consistently has average earnings of about £9k/month.

He's now had his child of course. His time is leveraged and he was able to bring in £10k the month that his son was born, even though he took 2 weeks off.

Adam realises this is a business model in which he can make the money he wants, while allowing him to have those months to take time off, look after his wife when she has just given birth and be at home to see their son grow up.

> It's a totally different conversation to how it was before; having little money, and the constant conflict between being around to support the family at home, versus working the long hours in the gym to earn the money.

Now, at the very top level, these people are making huge amounts of money and seeing incredible success. But the Insta-famous pro-card people who post 7 ab-selfies per day usually are not. They might have a fairly big following, but rarely is this translated in to actual business success.

They live and die by the validation they get from likes, but that doesn't translate to anything in the bank. They will have plenty of clients, but for the most part, they're in a similar position to everyone else – not enough hours in the day, charging by the hour and exhausted from trying to deal with so many different people.

This model of Insta-fame is like walking in to a mall with a machine gun, closing your eyes, pulling the trigger and spinning around in circles. You're going to get some hits, but there's a lot of wasted bullets.

Our coaching model is like a special-ops sniper. Lining up the head shot on the opposing general. Big bang for your buck, with little wasted effort.

Don't get us wrong, it's not that we are 'anti-fame'. There is a time and place for it, and often the people who are successful get it as a by-product of their success, not the cause.

You're looking for a high-quality lead to come in to your business. Someone who really needs your help and is most likely to buy. You don't need to care about everyone in the world seeing your material – most of them are never going to buy and will only waste your time.

This was one mistake that we made horribly in our previous failed business. We had bought in to the idea that building a big profile was the way to both appeal to the masses, and was a requirement to qualify yourself to the elite, high-paying, clients.

We had PR agencies, dozens of features in newspapers and magazines. Wrote our first book, including a big celebrity-filled launch party. We spent thousands on a beautiful website and professional high-quality videos.

We thought that image was everything. Any decision we took went through the filter of 'how will this be perceived?'.

We were more concerned about presenting a professional looking image and positioning ourselves in the right media, than we were about actually getting clients in to the business today.

It was all deferred to the future. After we do X, people will be banging our doors down.

Needless to say, this never happened. Every time something didn't go to plan, we moved the goalposts to the next thing, that was *sure* to be the answer.

It's tempting to look back and say we were doing anything to avoid selling, but honestly we didn't dislike selling. Like we mentioned earlier, we simply did not know that everything we were doing was stupid.

Nobody had ever told us that you need to do direct-response marketing, to get actual leads, and then sell to those people, to get clients. Nobody had told us that the lifeblood of any business is marketing and sales. Nobody had told us that *everything* else is useless without sales.

After all, with no sales, you have no clients to serve.

Direct-Response Marketing

We studied courses about business and even marketing, but it was the wrong kind of marketing. It was brand-building. Like what big companies with bottomless pockets do. 'Put our brand on TV 7,000 times and people will eventually remember it when they're looking for what we sell'.

That simply does not work for small businesses. It doesn't work for most big businesses either, but that's a different story.

It's all about perception. The big businesses are getting lots of exposure; shareholders see this and assume they must be doing well. That is what we were doing. We thought we were doing well because we had been featured in X place. We did everything apart from offer our services to our target market.

Instead of speaking to our potential clients who were right in front of us, we thought it was clever to build a profile and achieve a status that would let us get in to their company office, to speak to them all at once.

It's like we wanted a big bank to do our marketing for us. Clearly that was never going to work, but at the time it seemed like exactly the right thing to do.

We do think perception is changing on this, since Facebook ads became the hot new thing in fitness, people are starting to do direct-response marketing.

Whether Facebook is the right platform to do that or not, at least people are trying to generate leads and clients with direct-response marketing.

Direct- Response Marketing

Direct-response marketing is any form of marketing that is directly measurable, where you are asking the prospect to take a specific pre-determined action.

Buy, apply, join my email list, etc.

Direct response is measurable, because you are asking for a specific response, you can track how many people are taking that action.

Versus 'brand building' like you will see on TV or in magazines where companies have adverts that do not give any specific next step. These kinds of ads work to raise awareness, but they cost a fortune and are only appropriate for large companies with huge budgets.

As small businesses, our marketing needs to be measurable and accountable to an outcome, otherwise we are essentially throwing money down the drain.

It's funny looking back now, if we had known half of what we know about marketing back then, and had put all that money in to traffic instead of PR and pretty websites, logos and videos, we might just have been wildly successful.

But then we wouldn't be where we are now, and probably wouldn't be writing this book, so I guess learning the hard way has its benefits.

Why are we writing this book, by the way? Doesn't that go against what we are saying?

We are not anti-profile building. Being an author does build authority and it is a great front-end lead generator. Everyone else is writing blog posts or making YouTube videos. A full-length book is definitely a differentiator, but that's not really the point.
We have our marketing channels nailed down, where we can reliably generate leads as we need them. Now we have the freedom and time to spend writing a book, to pass off some of our knowledge to you and help you not make the mistakes that we did.

The first book that we wrote – I wouldn't call it a mistake – but we did it for the wrong reasons and did not make the best use of it.

For starters, it's a bad market to be writing in. The competition for female fitness and weight loss books is about as stiff as it can get.

It was a good experience and we did benefit from it, but we failed to make best use of it. It's funny, we spent 6 months writing and editing. Finding a publisher, agonizing over the name and cover art.

When it was finally released, we had a big (expensive) launch party… and proceeded to immediately forget all about the book.

We thought that having a book was the sole point, and moved on to doing other things. Like anything else, a book will not take off without marketing. Just having it sitting on Amazon will not get you much attention. We sell a couple of copies a month, but it hasn't even paid back the money we spent on it.

Well, maybe that's not true. In a roundabout way, it has, because we use it in our marketing channels. Giving away free copies, etc. and even just one client signing up would pay off the cost of getting it published (at least the financial cost, not the time and opportunity cost).

The point is, doing things like writing books is great when you are established and have an audience who want to hear from you. It is not a good way to build an audience.

At the beginning, you need to focus solely on generating leads and clients, with direct-response marketing.

Fame Does Not Equal Money

What to Do If You're Known in Your Gym/Area but Do Not Have a Following Online

Doing really well in your gym or local area, and maybe even fully booked…

But don't have a following online or know where to get online clients from?

Go to http://theprosperouspt.com/bonus to discover how to get started online, even if you have no profile whatsoever.

Here's a couple of stories to bring this point home.

What do you think would happen if you got a full double-page spread in the Sunday Times Business section?

Even better, with a great (if slightly crass) positioning headline that said something along the lines of "Elite Personal Trainer Charges £2,000 per Month".

Including a full picture and link to website. You could not ask for a better piece of publicity. Incredibly positioned, in the perfect media for the kind of high-end clientele that we were looking for. What happened?

A grand total of two (2) people got in touch. Of those two people, one was a time waster. The other was an assistant, on behalf of the very high-profile CEO of a huge company. We had some back and forth, but it ultimately didn't happen.

18 months later we sent her a copy of our book when it was published, to try and reignite the lead, and she did get in touch a while after that. She was busy travelling but we eventually came to an agreement that we were going to work together, in 3 months' time, when she was settled in London and had some consistency.

Anyway, a couple of weeks before we were due to start I got in touch and was told that she had changed her mind and it never ended up happening. Over 2 years of chasing up the one (1!) actual lead that came from this near perfect piece of publicity and it ended with nothing.

Even had she signed up, one client – worse, only one lead – is not a replicable system. We couldn't go and do that every week.

Another example of how this method doesn't work. For 18 months, I had my own column in Square Mile magazine. This is the biggest magazine in the City of London. A huge circulation to *all the right people*. Every month I had a full-page with an article about fitness and details of how to get in touch with me.

How many clients did I get from this? A grand total of...zero.

These things do help indirectly, they offer authority when you shout about them, but they are not a system for getting clients. Really that authority isn't even necessary when you know how to communicate to your perfect client and can sell effectively.

That's lots of talk about what not to do, and a nice exploration of our many failings. I imagine you're wondering what on earth does work?

What is direct-response marketing and how can I use it to get new clients in my fitness business?

Alright, let's look in to that.

5 MARKETING YOUR HIGH-VALUE ONLINE PROGRAM

Direct-response marketing is where you are taking the reader on a pre-determined set of steps to go from cold lead, to getting in touch with you. Giving specific instruction to do something; such as submit their email address, call you, or apply for a program.

The main thing is that direct-response marketing is within your control. You choose the media; you choose the action steps you want someone to take and you can scale it up as you choose.

A big piece of PR is great, but you have no control over it. You can't do it every day. When (if) it works, you can't just decide to do more of it.

Now, the problem for most trainers is that they don't have any active lead generation in place at all. You have some passive tools, like a website, but this relies on someone stumbling upon it on Google. You have no control over how many people are going to do this, or when.

Tim was making a fair amount of money as a PT. Yet he still had absolutely no way of getting a new client when he wanted.

It sounds appealing to have lots of money coming in from one person, but it is not a good business. If one person can leave and it instantly takes your business from thriving to struggling, that is not a good place to be. You know that every client is going to leave eventually.

Not wanting to beat a dead horse, but we should revisit why the old model of Personal Training is broken (again). If you're selling '10-blocks' of sessions for £500 or whatever, you have an unreliable business model that will not scale.

How much money can you spend to generate a client?

Not very much if they are only worth £500 to you, when you also consider gym fees and everything else that you have to spend to service that client.

The minimum possible value of a client using the new model is £2,000. When you look at upsells and continuation after the initial 12-week package, the average client value doubles to £4,000. If you know the average client value is £4,000 and your costs to service that client are basically zero, you can easily spend £100 to acquire a client if need be.

Let's not get ahead of ourselves though. You don't need to pay for leads just yet. There are 10's of thousands of pounds of untapped value in your business that you can get quickly and easily, for free.

You should start here and only consider paid ads when you have exhausted these channels.

Hierarchy of Lead Potential

This hierarchy explains where you should look for your leads. Go through it in order. It starts with the lowest hanging fruit – those who are most easily accessible and most likely to buy. You don't need to make generating leads harder than it needs to be. Start with the easiest ones first.

1. **Old clients** – Clients leave for a variety of reasons. Assuming you're good at what you do, it is probably not because they don't like your service or think that you are rubbish. Old clients can and do come back to work with you again, especially if you have a new service to offer that better meets their needs.

   Get in touch with all your old clients, tell them about what you are doing now and see if they would like to chat about it. We have both regained old clients (at much higher price points) by doing this.

   These people already know you, they already like and trust you. The situation that made them leave might not be the case now.

Maybe they moved away? Now you're online and you can work together again!

The worst that is going to happen is they aren't interested in chatting about your new services, but still appreciate you checking in on them, to see how they are going.

You should reach out to old clients once every 3 months and see if they want to jump on board.

2. **Existing clients (up-sell, cross-sell)** – If ever someone was likely to spend money with you, it is the people who are already doing so.

   You don't need to be 'salesy' about this. You're not trying to scam as much money as possible out of them, you are offering them a better level of service, which will help them to achieve their goals.

   If you have something good, that genuinely helps people, and you don't offer them it – is that not worse than if you did?

   You can up-sell PT clients or group training clients to coaching. A percentage of people will take you up and start spending more with you.

   You get to offer them a better service and help them even more, while growing your business.

   Again, don't just ask once but do so periodically. Especially if an existing package is coming to an end. Perhaps they have achieved the goals they set out to achieve? Well, I guarantee they will quickly have a new goal that you might be able to help them with.

   People are rarely satisfied for long and as soon as we have achieved one thing, we're looking ahead to the next goal.

3. **Referral** – Most PT's are not very good at generating referrals from their clients. Tim got a referral for a client worth £3,300/month from a £2,000/month client. How? He asked and then followed it up. It's not much more complicated than that.

   Most people will ask and then leave it there. Realise that clients are busy; they have things going on in their lives. They're not your full-time sales person. That said, they do want to help you, and they will do so.

What you need to do, is be consistent. Ask them and then make a point to follow it up with them. When they say, they might know someone, say something like;

"Cool, is it OK with you if I follow up on this in a week?".

They will say yes and then you follow them up in a week. Keep doing so, as many times as it takes.

It was at the 2nd reminder that Tim got this referral, which was worth a lot of money to him.

Ask your clients once a month if they know anyone who might benefit. People go through different phases of their life and in one moment a person can go from disinterested, to very hot to buy.

Something happens; they get dumped or have a health scare, and suddenly their body is number one priority. Keep asking clients and as their network go through different phases of life, they will find more people who might be appropriate.

Another example, one of the coaches in Tim's coaching group sent all his current clients a Christmas card with a referral gift card in it. He was the only person who followed through on this strategy and implemented it. Guess what? He got a £2,000 client from it.

The client who referred their friend even said thankyou to him!

You have to make it easy for them and follow it up. Be consistent and it will happen. Most trainers don't follow up and don't ask more than once. The chances are it's going to happen on the third, fourth, fifth time you ask. Keep checking in periodically.

4. **People who have contacted you for help or about your services, but never bought** – These people are obviously interested in your services. Just because, for whatever reason, they did not buy at that time, doesn't mean they will never buy.

Perhaps they were just not mentally ready to make the commitment back then, or maybe something happened since which has made it a higher priority. Phil had been loosely speaking to a lady for about 2 years and she had almost signed up a couple of times, but never did.

He followed her up a further time and it turned out she had got engaged earlier that month. Suddenly her situation had changed and she signed up straight away. This wouldn't have happened if he didn't keep in touch periodically.

5. **Anyone you've spoken to before** – The final place in the hierarchy goes to anyone you have interacted with before. They might not be as hot to buy as the people above, but they do have things going for them.

   Namely, they (hopefully) already know, like and trust you. This makes them a much more receptive prospect than a cold lead. It's less work to get them to a position of being ready to buy, because a brand new cold lead has to go through that know, like, trust phase anyway.

The Best Alternative Source of Clients If You Do Not Have a Big Email List

What if you don't have a big email list?

Or even any email list at all?

How can you find online clients? Is it going to take months? Will you have to pay for ads?

Go to http://theprosperouspt.com/bonus to discover the best alternative source of clients if you do not have a big email list.

There's a famous quote from legendary marketer Jay Abraham that says there are 3 ways to make more money in a business:

- Acquire more customers
- Increase the transactional value of each customer
- Increase the frequency of customer transactions

Everyone tends to focus on the first one, while neglecting the latter two. If you can up-sell existing clients, your business will grow. Without you having to spend the time, effort and money acquiring new customers.

This greater service of existing clients also tends to lead to them getting better results and having a longer, stronger relationship with you. Thus, being more likely to refer to you, giving you better case studies and proof elements - like before & after photos - to use in your marketing.

What about if someone you are training is not getting great results?

Perhaps because they only see you once or twice per week, or they're simply not following your advice outside of the gym.

Most trainers would fear having this conversation, because they're worried about losing the client, if they're not seeing results.

In our experience, clients almost always blame themselves for not seeing results. They know that they are not adhering to the advice you give them or working hard enough in the time away from you.

By actually offering them the help that they need to get results, you are doing them a favour. The person who is spending (wasting) money on training and isn't getting anywhere, because they don't follow the plan outside of the gym, is a prime prospect for coaching.

Phil had a group training client that, in 18 months, had lost a grand total of about 2kg. She liked the classes and had got fitter and stronger, but didn't follow the advice outside of the gym.

While she was very happy and a lifelong customer, she still had 15kg to lose and wasn't making progress. Probably kidding herself that, because she was training, she was 'trying'. Rationalizing it with excuses about genetics or metabolism.

He up-sold her to an online group coaching program (that was 5x the price) and she proceeded to get incredible results. Losing all the weight and completely changing who she was in relation to her body, exercise, food, etc.

This is one of my proudest success stories, because of how completely she has changed her life, and her partner's too. He also lost a similar amount of weight, and they both started doing CrossFit, fell in love with it and are now people who will be fit and healthy for life.

She knew she wasn't getting results – and she knew why – offering to help her in the area she needed it was the best thing I could do for her.

Always Follow Up

Perhaps you spoke to somebody last week and they were a 6/10 on how important it was for them to lose weight. Since then, they've been on a business trip and flew with Southwest Airlines in the US. When you fly Southwest, someone at the ticket counter will look at you, and if they determine you are too large to fit in the seats, they make you buy 2 tickets.

Can you imagine being at the airport and, for the first time, someone at the ticket counter is telling you that you're too fat for the seat and need to buy two tickets? In front of a queue of people. Having to pay twice the price for the flight.

Imagine the embarrassment and the pain that causes.

Do you think they might move up the scale from a 6/10 to a 10/10 after an experience like that?

If you don't follow up with people consistently and keep in touch with them, you will never know. Meanwhile, somebody else will do (fitness is a competitive market, after all) and probably take their business. They're probably not even as good as you are.

Alright, now that you know how to generate leads, the next step is converting them to clients.

6 SELLING YOUR HIGH-VALUE BODY TRANSFORM PROGRAMS

Dirty place, we know, but you've been to McDonald's, right?

When you go up and place an order, the server takes your order and charges you for the meal. Is that person good at selling?

They managed to close you...

Of course they're not. You've walked in there with the sole intention of buying a meal. The person taking your order could very well have been a computer screen.

This is what it's like when someone finds your website or profile in the gym and comes to you, looking to buy Personal Training. This is 'don't stick your foot in your mouth'. All you have to do is not say or do anything stupid, and you're guaranteed to have a client.

This doesn't mean you're good at selling.

Now consider this…

If I have a nice car, let's say a Mercedes and I want to sell it. I can stick up a post saying it's for sale for £3,000 – do you think I will meet much resistance in selling that car?

Anybody with £3k in the bank will be scrambling to give me their money.

But what if I sell it at it's true market value of £50,000. Now do you think everyone with a wallet and a pulse is going to be scrambling to give me their money? Probably not, right?

The only people who are going to buy, are people who really want the car, and they're going to have some resistance to overcome.

It's scary parting with a lot of money, isn't it? You will know if you've ever bought a house, car, or something of high-value.

Guiding someone through the transaction for £50k is a very different proposition than for the hugely under-valued £3k, wouldn't you agree?

Selling high-value Body Transformations is a different kettle of fish to selling low-value personal training. With PT, you're selling something that people are already looking to buy. It's not difficult.

To Be Successful…

You need to know how to sell high-value services. Most people do not go out searching for a solution that costs thousands (a few do). Most will look for the cheapest and easiest solution first – a gym membership or diet book – proceed to fail, and each time they do, move themselves up the ladder for how much they're looking to spend, to fix their problem.

You need to help them see that all the cheap solutions are not going to work. They need to make deep, fundamental changes in several areas that simply following a diet is not going to give them.

The irony is, personal training starts off looking cheap, but seeing someone 2-3 times per week for a year quickly runs in to the thousands. They end up spending more and achieving less than in a 12-week transformation that covers everything they're going to need, to see guaranteed results.

It's your duty to help these people save their time and money, by buying the service that actually delivers the value that they need. To do this, you need to show them that this is the case. That the very best solution for them is what you are offering.

(If what you offer is not the very best solution for them, don't even bother making them an offer).

Objections?

How to Overcome the Number 1 Objection Affluent Clients Have Against Online Training

Discover the number 1 reason affluent clients <u>will not</u> sign up for your online training program…and how to overcome it.

Go to http://theprosperouspt.com/bonus to overcome the number 1 objection affluent clients have against online training.

Do you get price objections now, selling PT for £30/50/70 an hour?

Imagine what you will get if you're selling a £2,000 package. Are you confident that you can overcome them and help the client see the value, and the need for them to invest in fixing this problem, right now?

The biggest difference when selling high-ticket packages is that you must help the client see the value they are getting.

The way to do this, is to listen to, and understand, the person on the other end of the phone. In a good sales conversation, you should be talking 5-10% of the time and letting them talk the rest of the time.

A lot of people equate selling with what they see on infomercials or from a stage. While that sells in that setting, where the conversation is only ever one-way, and you must make every argument for them buying your product possible, with great enthusiasm - that is not how people want to buy.

I learnt this quote from one of my mentors, serial entrepreneur, self-made millionaire and sales guru, Dave Thomson;
"People love to buy, but hate being sold. When you are telling them something, you are selling. When they say something, it is the truth".

Your role, is to ask the right questions, and let them sell themselves on working with you.

If you're talking, you are not letting them sell themselves. Even if they end up buying, they will feel like they've been sold to – and if they are buying, it's because they were always going to buy regardless.

When did someone last sit and really listen to you? Let you spill your heart and talk about what's going on in your life, without looking to get the conversation back to themselves; just waiting for you to stop talking, so that they can start?

When did someone seem genuinely interested in what you were saying, and encourage you to go deeper and expand on what you're saying?

We call the role that you play in a sales call the 'interested introvert'. Now, that may or may not be your natural personality, but when you're in a sales conversation, it is one that you should adopt.

To listen to what they are saying and be genuinely interested in hearing it. What happens, is people will have breakthroughs, just by you asking the right questions and keeping them talking.

Transformation Happens in The Sale

The sales conversation is probably the single most important part of someone's transformation. On the call, they – for the first time ever – will see just how important this is for them, they will honestly assess why they are in the situation that they are in, and what needs to change for them to move forwards.

Their eyes will be opened to the reality of the matter, with your help. On a successful call, they will not only see the truth of the situation (which is a requirement for them to succeed), but they will also make the commitment to changing.

They will admit that they need help and by putting (a significant amount of) their money in to it, they are going 'all in'. They're making the commitment that they have never made before.

Every other time, they can (and do) back out when things get hard. Inevitably, there will be times on the journey when someone struggles.

Their brain revolts at the idea of change. Their self-image and perception doesn't believe that they are the healthy, slim person they want to be, and will do everything it can to self-sabotage them.

Every other time, this is when they quit. They get frustrated, and quietly crawl back in to their shell. This time is different, because they have made that commitment to getting help. They've put their money in to it, and losing that will be more painful than the pain of change.

This simply does not happen when someone is paying a small amount, or paying the investment off over time. A large, upfront payment is a statement of intent. It's their commitment that they are doing this and cannot back out.

Now, they probably won't see it like that in the heat of the moment, but that is the reality and it is your duty to help them. You have to make them commit to a permanent change, and that comes during a good sales conversation.

You don't sell to them, and then start working together. The selling *is the first 50% of their transformation.*

Sell by Listening…

When someone knows that you understand their problem, they naturally assume that you have the solution. You do not need to tell them that you have the solution, let them come to their own conclusions on that. Your role is simply to understand their problem, and to show them that you understand it.

Listen, probe, repeat what they say back to them, and go on a journey together, exploring their problems. Nobody will have ever done this with them before; you will be head and shoulders above anybody else – you don't need to justify why you're so much more expensive. You are simply playing a completely different sport.

A Personal Trainer or a diet club is not a comparison to what you do.

"What's the best way to get good at sales?"

You can and should study the act of selling. You need to understand the process and how to do it. Following a 'script' doesn't work very well, but you should have a 'journey' outline that you follow.

We use the 6-step selling system; Open > Pain > Pleasure > Bridge > Close > Objections.

Once you have this, the only way to get good, is to get on the phone and speak to people. Speak to as many people as you possibly can. You learn by doing. Only experience and getting a feel for how the other person reacts is going to lead to improvement.

The biggest struggle we see people having is a reluctance to get on the phone and get rejected 10 times on the trot. People are too tied up in the outcome and attach their worth to the person's answer.

You should view these conversations as practice. You have to believe that the right clients will say yes and the wrong clients for you will say no. This is a good thing, if you did try and work with the wrong client, they wouldn't get results anyway, because you're not a fit for each other.

Over time, you start to know who the right clients are, and you will spend less time speaking to people who are not a fit. Your conversion rates will go up at this point. Until then, until you have the experience of speaking to dozens and dozens of people, you have no right to expect it to all be plain sailing.

You have no right to assume that high-level sales are easy and you should get it right immediately. That's a ridiculous notion. You must pick up the damn phone and get rejected over, and over again. Until you do, you simply cannot be good at sales.

You will remain an 'order taker', like your chap at McDonald's. You can kid yourself that someone is coming and paying you money, so you must be good at sales – but you will never move to the level where you can genuinely help all the people who most need your help.

You will remain at the whim of your clients, and never have the control to build the business that you desire.

Qualifying

"So the answer is just talking to as many people as possible?"

Prior to speaking to them, you should be qualifying the people you speak to. The better you understand your avatar and perfect client, the more you can qualify them. The more you will only speak to the people who are a good fit.

Before doing a sales call, we recommend that you have a process for qualifying people. Bridge the gap between them reaching out, and you being ready to get on the phone with them. You want to know that they are a qualified, serious prospect who needs your help, and is potentially ready to invest.

This process achieves a number of things:

- It protects your time and you don't spend an hour on the phone with someone who is just not serious about making a change
- It makes them qualify to you. Making you harder to access and thus perceived as valuable
- Each interaction builds commitment, allowing them to know, like and trust you, and be more ready to do business with you
- Sets the scene for what will happen in the consultation, so they feel comfortable with the process

Let them know that you are going to help them by looking at where they are now, where they want to be and after that, looking at what they need to overcome to get there. Then you will make a plan to do so. This has huge value to the client, whether they sign up to work with you or not.

Let them know that IF you think you are a good fit for each other, and that you can help them, you will make them an offer. If not, you won't. Get their permission to do this and it doesn't feel 'salesy'. Like we said before, people love to buy, but hate being sold.

Sales = BAD?

Let's change gear for a minute. Tell us, when we say 'sales' – what words come to mind?

There's a famous study that showed on average, of the first 20 words people thought, 19 had negative connotations.

19 out of 20!
People are uncomfortable with sales. They think of the sleazy used car salesman. They're indoctrinated by media, parents, teachers, that sales are bad, dirty, and sleazy. That money is the root of all evil.

People fear losing money, they've bought things before and had a negative experience, which left a bad feeling. They have the psychological baggage of their parents, telling them money doesn't grow on trees, and that they shouldn't spend it on themselves.

If you feel like this yourself, you will not be successful. Ever.

You might start to see success, but you will sabotage yourself. You will not keep pushing forwards if your belief patterns about money and sales are negative.

You're going to have to do some introspection and overcome these. Change your beliefs. Just like helping the client change their belief about their body, their self-image, and halting their sabotaging behaviours. You must do the same with money.

On the client side, they probably have the same shit going on in their head. You need to use the power of persuasion to get them to a position where they are comfortable enough to spend money on something that they desperately want and need help with.

Persuasion and influence often get a bad rep. You must recognise that they are tools. You can use a hammer to build a house for your family, or you can bash someone over the head with it. The hammer is not inherently good or evil. It is simply a tool that you use to achieve an outcome.

Sales, persuasion and influence is the same. Nothing changes in the world without a sale being made. It is your duty to learn how to move people to action, and to use it in an ethical way.

Why You Should Always Charge Top Prices

The argument for high prices: when someone invests at a stretch, they really mean it. They are committed and serious about making changes, and there is a genuine financial downside that is going to sting, if they do not do what they've committed to doing. Not always, but the vast majority of times.

Have you ever had 2 clients that are a similar size, age, job, personality, etc. One person does what you say and gets amazing results. The other gets absolutely nowhere. What's the difference?

The only difference is the *implementation*.

The value you have provided is the same. The information you give is just as good. The recommendations just as well-thought out and appropriate.

The only variable, is what the client does with it. The sale, and eventually the transformation, is a meeting of your service and the client's implementation. Without implementation; you can know everything there is to know, have the perfect plan for someone, the answer to every problem.

It is zero use, without their implementation.

Where somebody meets you in the market, is the value of your product. If someone comes in and pays £50, they value your service at £50. If someone comes in and pays £2,000, they value your service at £2,000.

Who is going to get better results? The person who values your service more! Same information, same service. Different level of commitment, different level of implementation.

By being cheap, you are doing your clients a disservice. It does not help them by making it 'affordable'. That is just making them less committed and less likely to follow through on it.

"But fitness should be free for everyone".

It is. Join a library, get a book out, follow it. Or Google, follow the advice on any decent plan and you'll get results. People choose, for whatever reason, NOT to follow it. They want help doing so, and of course they have to invest to get that.

Think about it like this - if I want to paint my house, I can do it myself, or if I want someone to help me with it, I'll pay a decorator - I don't complain that painting and decorating services aren't freely available to all.

When you become successful in your business, bring in enough income in to comfortably support yourself and your family, you can free up time, then go and offer your knowledge for free to people.

But to be blunt the people who, in our experience, say fitness should be free/cheap fear selling, rejection, and even making too much money.

What the Client Thinks...

What sort of client do you want to work with? The one who comes in and implements at a £2k value, or the one who implements at a £50 value?

No-brainer, right?

The better client to work with, the one who gets better results and takes the whole thing seriously, is the one who has invested significantly.

What if you think you're not worth that amount of money?

"Won't clients turn their nose up at it?"

Some will, but they're not the people who need your help. They don't value it enough. The pain is not great enough for them to be committed and invest in a transformation, at that level.

When your clients do take your plans, and implement on them, do they get results? Are they happy at the end?

If you asked them, do you think they would say they got good value? If the answer is yes, then you are worth the money!

I had a client, who admittedly was outrageously rich, but when we were having the sales conversation, I quoted him £12k (for 16 weeks) and he asked me if that was per month! People will pay what you ask them for.

At the end of his transformation, I asked him how much he would value it at now, and he told me it was easily worth £100,000 to him. It had changed his life so much, that he would have been happy to pay a six-figure sum for it.

Obviously, this is relative, most people *don't have a six-figure sum to spend, on anything.* The point is the value that he got from it was 10x my already very high prices.

The most important step in this whole process, is the initial sale. You are setting the value that the client is going to attach to their transformation. The greater the fee that they buy in at, the greater value they perceive their transformation to be worth. The greater the value, the more seriously they will take it.

When someone pays up-front they're subconsciously in it for the long run. If they're paying monthly, or worse, for sessions, they can drop out at any time.

There will come a point when they are facing resistance and self-doubt. Their brain throws a hissy-fit because their self-image is not that of someone who is in great shape and does these behaviours you are recommending.

Motivation drops and excuses start to pile up. It is the natural human reaction to change. You will have to fight through this to make changes in any area of life. You don't want your clients to have an easy back out.

You want them to work through it, with your support. Instead of them hiding away and avoiding you when they are in this resistance – the time that they most need your help – you want them coming to you for support.

How Should You Be Pricing Yourself?

If almost everyone that you speak to is signing up at your current price point, it is too cheap.

"But aren't I helping more people if they all sign up?"

No, you're not, because you are not filtering for the people who *really* need your help.

When you put the prices up, only the people most in need of your help are going to commit, and that is a good thing. You're going to have a bigger impact and your clients are going to all experience greater transformation.

You'll also find that you generally weed out all the clients who are hassle to work with, who challenge you and don't follow through on what you've advised them to do. Remember, your effectiveness is the meeting of your information, with their implementation.

Tim's coaching client started off selling semi-private PT sessions at £997 for 12 weeks (he was offering a combo of online and offline). At this price point he had an incredibly high closing rate, so he kept putting his prices up and up. To £1,200, then £1,500. To £2,000 and ultimately up to £2,000 for 8 weeks, instead of 12.

He met almost no resistance throughout this process. He just kept getting better, more committed clients and his business grew and grew. He could let most of his PT clients go, as their packages came to the end, and focus just on helping more high-value clients online.

Conversion Rates

You'd think converting every sales call into a client is good, right? In fact, 80% or above conversion rates are not what we are looking for. It means you are not pushing hard enough, and your prices are too low. You will be taking on people who are not fully committed, or not really in need of your help.

Totally different to most people, who are trying to close 1 out of 1 and get dejected when they fail. The best clients, who most need your help and are fully committed, will invest in a high-value program.

Of course, you need to have the lead generation to have plenty of people to talk to. This is what keeps most people stuck, not working with their dream clients. They simply are not doing the marketing to have enough leads to choose from.

To sell like this, where you're almost looking for the rejection, you must remain unattached to the outcome.

You want to help people, but if someone doesn't commit, it is not a reflection of your value or ability, it is a reflection of their pain and desire. It's just not important enough for them, and that's ok.

"What does a sales call look like?"

The basic overview of a sales call looks like this:

Where are you now? > Where do you want to be? > What stops you getting there? > Objection handling > Close

Throughout this process you should be sitting back and listening the vast majority of the time. The client should do 90% of the talking, and they should be selling themselves on working with you.

You have this structure in your mind, of the way a conversation flows and you are guiding it there. Don't let the client de-rail it by going off on tangents, feeling the need to answer their questions about things, if the timing is not right, or it is not important.

The right answer to a question is always another question. When they ask you something, you flip it back and ask them.

Why? Because when you tell them something, you are selling. When they tell you something, it is true.

Energy Transfer

There is an energy exchange in a sales call. One person will be controlling the energy and the other person will be qualifying to them. Most people are trying to 'sell themselves'. They're trying to convince the other person as to why you should work together.

This is the wrong way around, and it is not an effective way to sell. You should be controlling the energy and have the client qualifying themselves to you. They're selling themselves on working with you, remember. Your role is to facilitate them doing that. Trying to do it for them does not work.

Nobody likes to be sold to, and everyone is put off when they are 'pitched'. However, people do like to buy. Let them convince themselves, and it will never feel pushy or uncomfortable. It is an enjoyable process.

You want to get to a position where the client is selling themselves to you. Where you are genuinely only going to make offers to the right people and they need to show you why they are going to be a good client. Why you should let them in to your program, and agree to help them.

I remember on one call; I wasn't sure about someone. I asked her what type of client she was going to be. She started to sell herself to me, telling me how good she would be to work with, how important it was, how she would do everything I asked her. I did make her an offer in the end, I said "Ok, I will accept you in the program" and she cheered. No joke, cheered, out loud, the fact that I would let her pay me 2 grand.

Can You Sell?

Sales is one of those things that everyone thinks they can do. Nobody thinks they're bad at selling. To be honest, that's not a bad thing. Confidence is super important in selling.

To *really* get good at sales, you need to be accountable to the numbers.

Record your calls and improve the process. Listen back to them and see where you have let the energy slip, and started qualifying to them.

Make notes and record your numbers. You should know how many people you need to speak to, on average, to make a sale. It will be pretty consistent. If you improve over time it will change, but it is not totally random.

Detach Yourself

One of my clients was a model, she was slim, but as models go, she wasn't quite as thin as the average. She would go to castings and when she was carrying a little bit too much body fat, would get people literally come up to her, grabbing hold of her fat. Talking about how she was a bit too fat, openly, in a room full of 30-40 other models who were at the casting.

Can you imagine how embarrassing and painful that experience would be?

Yet, she loved modelling so much, it gave her such satisfaction when she was on the job, that she would never give it up.

She was working on being leaner, but wanted to remain healthy. She refused to use the 'cigarettes and cocaine diet' that most of her peers were on, to remain so skinny.

She had to learn to become unattached to the casting decision. That her self-worth was not attached to someone's opinion of whether she was 'too fat'.

It's the same when you are selling. You want to help people – just like she wanted the modelling job – but you have to detach and remain unaffected when you get rejected. You cannot take it to heart and let it impact the way you interact with the next potential client.

People often choose not to get your help because they don't trust or believe *in themselves*. It's often not anything about you. They simply lack confidence in their own ability to do this.

This comes naturally when you attain a certain level of success. When business is predictable and paying you handsomely, you begin to develop an abundance mindset, and genuinely do not need any one client to sign up.

To get there, you're going to have to do the hard work. You will have to push through the resistance and commit to doing the work, whatever happens.

That is the same relationship we have with clients. For the most part, you can tell them what to do in an hour or two, and if they take that and implement, they will be successful. So, why do they need you after that?

They need the support and accountability to implement on what they know. They need a push to get them to do something that they do not 'want' to do. That is most of what we do as trainers and coaches, we act as the little angel on their shoulder, ensuring that they walk the right path.

Realistically, you are not giving your clients a great deal of information every time you speak, after the first couple of weeks. They know what to do, they just need the help to actually do it. You're an implementation facilitator.

Objections to Making Offers

Trainers come up with all sorts of reasons to not get out there, have sales conversations and make offers to would-be clients.

We used to be guiltier of this than anyone, as you can see from our journey getting to this point.

Here's some of the things we will hear people saying is stopping them getting on the phone, making offers and sales. This is not a judgement by the way; we did most of these ourselves for years:

- Need a website
- Need to 'create the program' first
- Logos
- Business cards
- Making/editing videos
- Writing mission statements
- Building social media following
- 'Giving value' before trying to make sales

None of this is necessary or even helpful. It's busywork that distracts you from the actual goal of making sales and helping clients. It's a back-out; to not have to get on the phone with potential clients and face possible rejections.

What we recommend. What we both did when we *actually got somewhere* is we sold the program first. We got out of our own way and launched it. Then created it in real time as it was delivered.

Sell First, Create Later

When you are coaching in the style that we recommend, there really is no 'program'. It is 100% unique and individual. Totally based on the situation each different client is presenting, each week.

This is why you need higher level skills, to know what is going on and react correctly. To be able to take the 10,000-foot view, see what is happening and the right course of action, but also be able to bring that back to earth in the client's language. Giving them one or two simple things to implement which will make all the difference.

You cannot hide behind a pre-written training program.

How to Start Your Online Business If You're Fully Booked in Person & Have No Free Time

Fully booked in your in-person business?

Great! Of course, it does present a small problem if you want to go online – a lack of free time.

Go to http://theprosperouspt.com/bonus to discover how to start your online business, even if you have no time because you're fully booked in person.

In Tim's mentorship, he offers 'The £2k, 12 Week Results Blueprint' training module, explaining exactly how to coach people. There are milestones you want to get clients to, but it naturally has to be flexible and individualised.

Realise that when you are doing basically anything other than selling or delivering services, it is avoidance. Nothing else is going to take you forwards.

Down the road, perhaps creating systems and a nice website might help – though that is debatable – but at the start it is the wrong thing to do. You don't even know if anyone wants to buy your stuff yet. Don't waste 6 months putting everything in place to find that out down the road.

Get on the phone, speak to as many people in your market as possible, and make offers. Don't reject yourself by projecting on to other people that they will not want your help.

It's easy to tell yourself that they can't afford it or they won't want your help, but until you ask, you don't know this to be the case. If the problem is big enough for someone, they will spend money to fix it.

£2,000 for an online program sounds like a lot, but your PT clients spend that much with you over 3-4 months anyway. The fact it is paid upfront and delivered remotely doesn't make the actual amount of money greater. It is going much further, in terms of generating results for the client.

One of Tim's earliest clients trained with him for £45 an hour. The very same lady went on to spend £8,000 (£2,000 on a 12-week program, then £6,000 on a 12-month Mastery program) on coaching. People can and do spend the money *when they see the value*. Again, people will meet you at the value that you present yourself.

If you come to market at a £45 value, people will pay £45. If you meet the market at £2,000 value, people will pay £2,000!

What if you don't know what to do? How to deliver this? How to do sales?

The only way to find out, is to do. No amount of thinking about it is going to come close to doing it. Get on the phone and speak to people. The more people you speak to, the more you will understand what people need.

Will you get rejected a lot at first? Possibly. View it as research. Every conversation is helping you to understand what people need your help with. Soon you will have a picture of what people do and do not need from you. That is what you deliver.

This might sound a bit wishy-washy, but ultimately it is individualisation. Going back over it again, this is why you must be a highly skilled and knowledgeable coach. You need to know all the information and be able to see through that complexity, to pluck out the simplicity - one or two big things that move the client forwards – and shelter them from all the bullshit that causes overwhelm and procrastination.

Often, you end up giving advice that a random on the street could have come up with.

"Drink more water and run around the block a couple of times this week".

The difference is, you understand that this is the level the client is at, as an individual and importantly, where they need to go next to progress.

Until you are actually coaching people and helping them. Having them go away and implement; then coming back with feedback – their results and what they have struggled with – you do not know what help they will need.

Guessing, and creating *stuff* because you equate it with 'value' is not helping. It is overwhelming and will make client outcomes worst, not better. Let the client's outcomes determine the help that they need, at each stage of the journey.

7 CONCLUSION

In a minute, we're going to give you a guide to get started today. First, let's briefly recap the main points, so they're fresh in your mind as you set off on your journey to becoming a highly paid, highly impactful online coach.

The old PT model is dying. You cannot continue to sell time for money, working long and unsociable hours for the rest of your life if you want more for yourself and your family. Further to this, the client doesn't get as much benefit or as good a service as they should get, when you follow this model.

Aside from the 1% of the population that are athletes or bodybuilders, people do not lack information or opportunity to get in shape. The problem isn't that people do the wrong diet plan or need to train 20% harder. The problem is that they simply don't do anything. At least not consistently.

As a coach, to impact these people you do not need to give them information, you need to help them action the information that they more than likely already know. The implementation brings results, and it is the results that people seek.

Nobody *wants* to hire a Personal Trainer – it's just the means to getting in shape. You are doing a better job by making this process easier, faster, simpler and more sustainable. That means giving the clients more responsibility, less information and more accountability.

You're going to have to step outside of the 'PT model' and shift your mindset to serve your audience at the highest level, and be rewarded for it.

The PT business does not work. You're more than likely proving that right now. Take your knowledge, your experience, your passion and apply it in a different model, one that allows you to have the freedom and security you strive for in your business.

The chances are, you're not going to be the next Body Coach. The costs are huge, and chance of failing overwhelming. The safer, reliable model is the high-priced coaching which is actually a higher level of service than Personal Training. You're giving your clients less time – but bigger results.

The business model is extremely simple and requires nothing to get started. Do not get bogged down in websites, social media and business cards. Simply work out your client avatar – the person you feel most pulled to serve – and start putting messages out to those people.

Marketing should be simple and direct, when you're targeting in on people and speaking directly to their problems, they will be happy to talk to you about helping them. Now you're on to closing the sale – the moment their transformation begins. You must do everything in your power to get a client on board, *if they are a fit and genuinely need your help.*

Once you have the client, the delivery is simple – this is the area you already excel in. You're ready to go ahead, get great results with your clients, have them refer their friends and start making a difference in the world.

That's all that is left to say. Go and start today.

8 HOW TO START TODAY

In this final section of the book we are going to give a brief outline of what you need to do first, to start today. The bonus material at http://theprosperouspt.com/bonus will support you doing this.

Access Our Little Black Book of Tools & Resources You Need to Start Online

Go to http://theprosperouspt.com/bonus for our list of ALL the tools and resources you need to run a successful online training business.

We have tried and tested many different tools, and this is the list of the best and ONLY the most necessary tools you will need.

Step 1

Decide on your avatar. The very first thing you must do is decide who you wish to work with. Until you know who you are going to work with, you cannot possibly create or market a program that is going to be suited for their needs, right?

Use the avatar exercise at http://theprosperouspt.com/bonus to establish exactly who you wish to serve.

Step 2

When you know who your service is for, you need to determine what their problems are. What is it you are going to help them with?

It's vital that you build your avatar out, even though we say start by speaking to current and past clients, who may not be your avatar.

You want to start with low hanging fruit – the people who already trust you. There is a small pool of these people, and once you have exhausted them, you need the depth and coherence that comes from marketing to a specific avatar. This will allow you to build that same level of trust quickly.

Step 3

Communicate to people based on their pains and desires – not based on what you do. Nobody cares what you do until you give them reason to care.

That reason being, you showing them that you understand the situation they are in, the problems they face and where they wish to get to. When you show them that you know this, they know that your service is the answer. You don't have to tell them.

These exercises should take no more than 1 hour in total. It's very important information to know, but it is only a starting point.

As you speak to more people and gain more experience within your market, you will come to have greater understanding of your prospect's life. You can continue to refine your avatar and targeting as your business progresses.

What you should not do, is use it as an excuse to procrastinate. You must move forwards, put something out to the market to get feedback and adjust from there. Without starting – which is what a lot of people do, spending weeks messing around with websites and logos – you don't have any true data. You are only guessing, wasting your time and not serving your audience.

Step 4

Now you know who you are looking for, where do you find them?

This is not a marketing book, but we are going to help you. This is the simplest, quickest, easiest and most effective way to find clients.

Reach out to the people already in your network. They are your hottest prospects. That means:

- Current clients
- Former clients
- Referrals
- People who had consults and didn't buy
- People who've asked advice or you have chatted with
- People on your email list or Facebook page

This is the lowest hanging fruit and where you should always look for your first clients.

When you are marketing, you are looking to *open a conversation*. Nothing more.

You're not trying to close a sale; you're simply opening a line of communication. The easiest way to do this when you begin, and don't yet have a program in place or much information about your audience, is simply to ask them.

Genuinely do research by reaching out to your audience, and asking what their struggles are, why they've failed before, where they need help, etc.

They will tell you exactly what they want to buy from you!

A shockingly high percentage will also be desperate to buy it from you. They will ask you if you can help, just because you're likely the first person to have reached out and listened to them.

Curiosity will take you a long way. Be curious and find out the information that is valuable to you be able to serve people to the best of your abilities.

A simple segue;

> *"Do you want to know when I've put the program together?"*

Will almost always get a positive response and allow you to transition into a sales call.

Some books might give you a script of exactly what to say here. We don't like scripts, they will work sometimes, but you are not learning anything, and the other person will almost always deviate off script in real life.

Like Mike Tyson says;

"Everyone has a plan, until they get punched in the face".

Coaching a client *always* has unexpected deviations from the 'perfect plan'. You must be prepared for this, and flexible in your approach to navigate these issues. Keeping the client's confidence and adherence high in these make-or-break moments when they have always fallen off the rails in the past.

This is simple. Don't think about it from a marketing perspective. Think from a human perspective. It's a normal conversation you would have with a normal person in a normal situation.

Re-engage them with a simple message such as;

> *"Hey NAME, I've finished putting together the initial stages of the [PROGRAM].*
>
> *I think it would really help you to [Achieve goal they told you]. Do you want to have a chat about it?"*

From there, just organize a time that works for both of you to jump on a call and talk about your new program.

Marketing like this is much simpler than you think. You're going to ask people what they struggle with. They're going to tell you. Then you can repeat it back in your marketing. Don't guess, ask.

Step 5

Sell your online program.

We recommend you charge £2,000 and that is the price that people in Tim's mentorship program begin selling their programs. It's proven successful, and is the right balance between being affordable, but enough of an investment that people are fully committed.

Now, depending on your background and how you feel about your service you might not be comfortable charging £2,000 right now.

If not, that's cool – not everyone can start off that that price. The people that have done are top coaches with lots of experience, and they've invested in the help and support of a coach to get them going on their online training journey.

Maybe you can't charge £2k off the bat, but you can definitely charge £1,000 for a 12-week transformation.

We strongly recommend you approach it with the idea that your program is £2,000 – but you're going to beta test it first. You can actually tell people that;

> *"This is a £2,000 program.*
>
> *I know my program works and 100% I will get you results. However, this is the first time I am running this specific program.*
>
> *Therefore, there will be some bumps along the way and you might have to bear with me from time to time.*
>
> *We will get you the results regardless, but because this is a new program I can offer you a first-time entry rate of just £1,000 if you commit now".*

Where do you value yourself?

If you value yourself at £2k, go right ahead and charge that. If not, the aim is to get to £2k. It's a proven price point by lots of people.

Realistically, to make this work at £2k you will probably need some help. Reading a book is like your client reading your blog, versus working with you in person.

They will get good information, and get some results if they action it – but you don't expect a few blog posts to take them all the way to where they want to be.

One important note, the value proposition must be relative, if you are going to start at a slightly lower price point. Clients must be committed. 'Testing' it at £200 is simply not the same thing. The price should be an investment that brings commitment from the client, and stretches you in delivering it.

After selling a couple of programs at £1,000 – or whatever price point you choose – put the price up.

"Once is an instance, twice is a co-incidence, 3 times is a law".

When you've sold 3 places, you can put your prices up. You have proven it works and that you can do it.

Congratulations!

You're awesome, you've read the entire book.

At the beginning of the book we talked about the difference between winning and losing. You've got to the end of the book, showing us that you're the kind of person who follows through.

Well done!

You're in the top 10% of committed action takers who are on course to become winners in the fitness industry.

The next step is for you to go to http://theprosperouspt.com/bonus and download the resources, to begin taking action today.

Use the final section of the book 'How to Start Today' as a workbook. Refer back to it as you implement these steps in your business and get your very first high-value online training clients.

Good luck and thank you for reading.

ABOUT THE AUTHORS

Tim Drummond and Phil Hawksworth are authors of an Amazon best-selling women's fitness book, featured in The Sunday Times, Hello Magazine and Daily Mail. They both work 100% online; Phil travelling the world, Tim spending his summers in London and winters in Spain.

Made in the USA
Charleston, SC
20 February 2017